ROXY/HORNBAKER

THE
SURF
GIRL
HAND
BOOK

Everything you need
to know about surfing
– and so much more!

SURFGIRL MAGAZINE
IN ASSOCIATION WITH ROXY

KATE CZUCZMAN

Published by Orca Publications
Berry Road Studios
Berry Road
Newquay
Cornwall
TR7 1AT
United Kingdom
(+44) 01637 878074
www.surfgirlmag.com
www.orcasurf.co.uk

EDITOR: **LOUISE SEARLE**
DESIGNER: **DAVID ALCOCK**
EDITORIAL CONSULTANTS: **STEVE ENGLAND AND ROB BARBER**
SUB-EDITOR: **ALEX HAPGOOD**
DISTRIBUTION CONSULTANT: **CHRIS POWER**
PRODUCTION: **MIKE SEARLE**

EDITORIAL CONTRIBUTORS: Alex Hapgood, Lucia Griggi, Joel Gray, Rowena Wilson,
Sarah Beardmore, Easkey Britton, Kirsty Jones, Rob Barber, Celine Gehret, Izzy Keene

PHOTOGRAPHIC CONTRIBUTORS: Mike Searle, Chris Power, Roger Sharp, Simon
Williams, Kate Czuczman, Alan Van Gysen, Dale Adams, Darrell Wong, Alex Williams

THE SURF GIRL HANDBOOK ISBN 978-0-9523646-1-0

PRINTED AND BOUND: **GREAT WALL PRINTING, HONG KONG**

SURFING CAN BE A DANGEROUS SPORT.

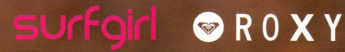

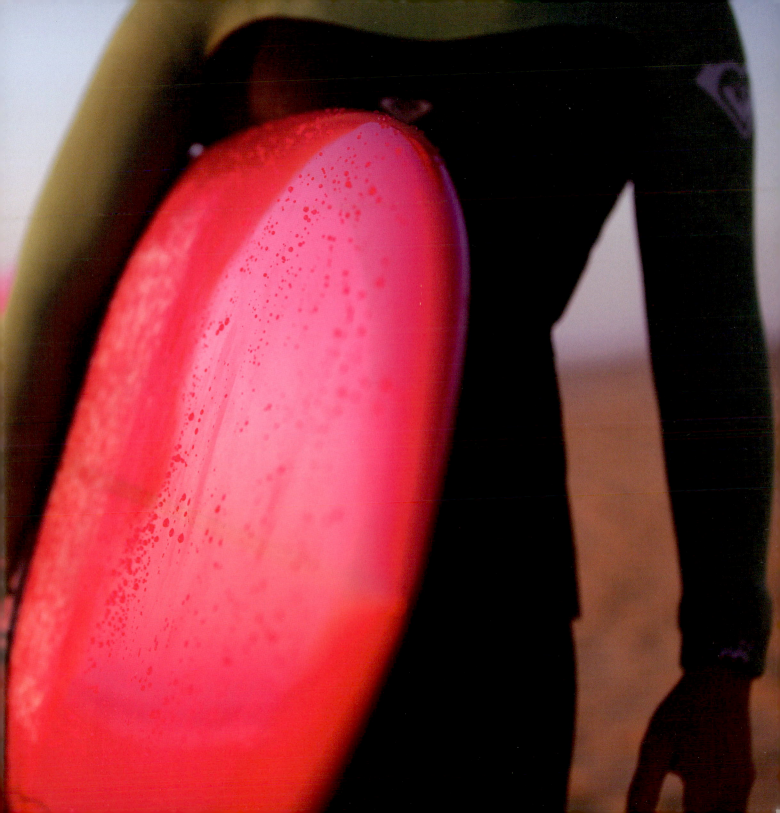

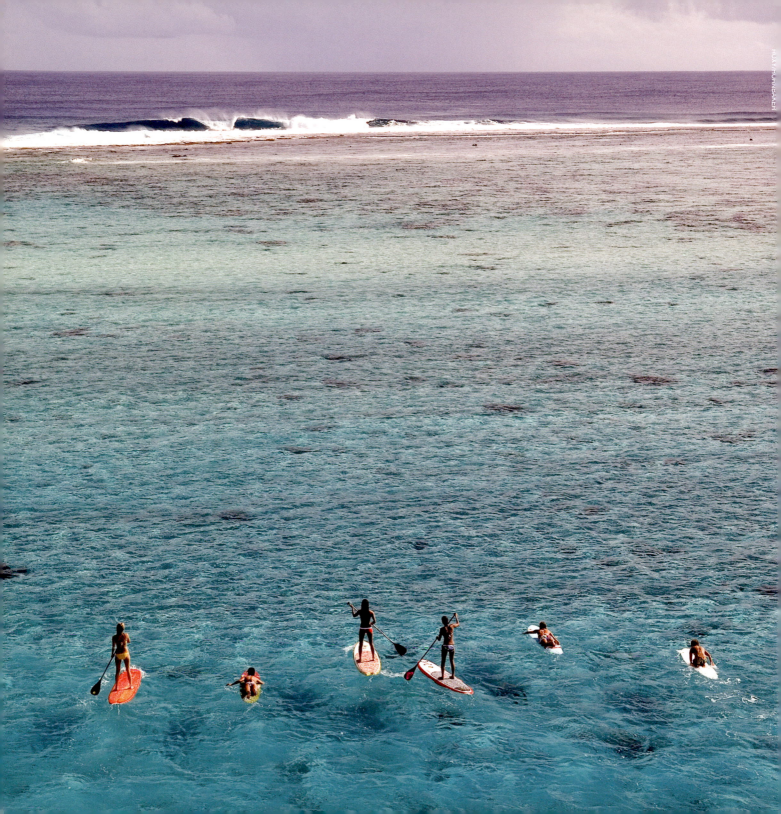

CONTENTS

FOREWORD

I was six years old when I learned to surf with my dad and three older brothers on a quiet south coast beach of New South Wales, Australia. It was a popular passtime for many families in our sleepy little town of Gerroa. Following in my brother's footsteps, it wasn't until I was eleven that I decided to turn my attention to competition. Millions of people surf today from all over the world for different reasons but very few end up making a competitive career out of it.

The Surf Girl Handbook provides an invaluable guide for the novice through to the semi pro surfer wanting some tips to take their surfing to the next level. The book isolates the key manoeuvres and breaks them down, offering just the right amount of guidance so as not to make it too confusing. The photos of the pro's performing manoeuvres gets the adrenaline pumping. The Surf Girl Handbook will inspire you to want to get out there and do it yourself.

I will have my love of surfing for my entire life. The elements of the ocean are forever changing and it always has you searching for that next perfect wave or perfect section and ultimately a perfect session. Surfing is something that I became hooked on, besides it being insanely fun, it provides that challenge which feeds my competitive hunger. The challenge of wanting to improve and continue to learn new manoeuvres every time I hit the water.

The Surf Girl Handbook is a definite read. I highly recommend reading as much quality information about your passion and then sorting through what applies to your level or style of surfing. I never turn down new information, it may just be the trigger you need for your next big breakthrough with what you're working on.

Never lose sight of the fun and enjoyment you gain just from being in the ocean and surrounded by mother nature.

See you all in the lineup!

Surfer for life,

Sally

SALLY FITZGIBBONS, PRO SURFER

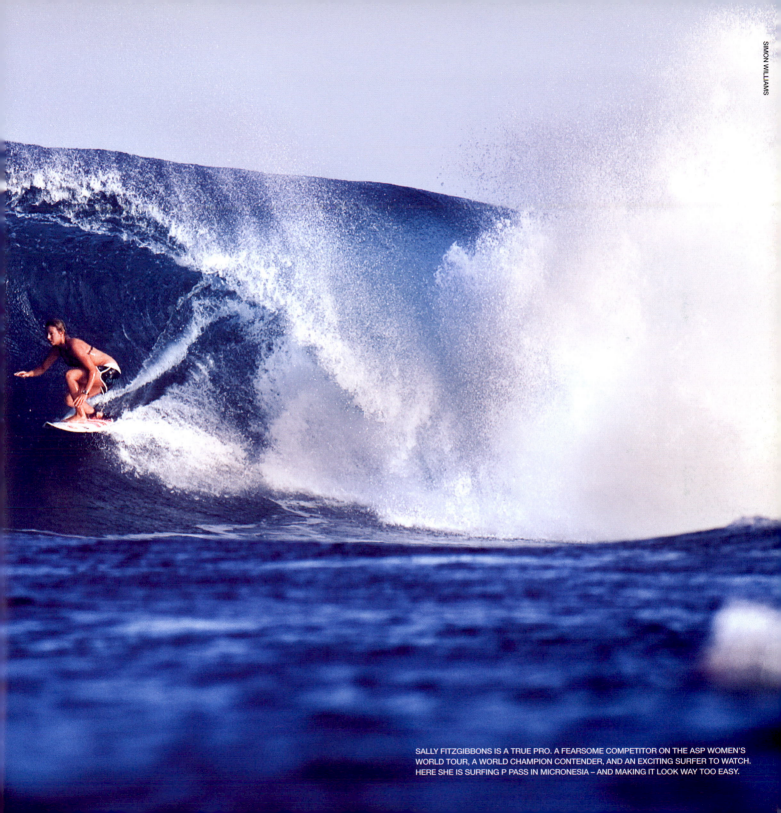

SALLY FITZGIBBONS IS A TRUE PRO. A FEARSOME COMPETITOR ON THE ASP WOMEN'S WORLD TOUR, A WORLD CHAMPION CONTENDER, AND AN EXCITING SURFER TO WATCH. HERE SHE IS SURFING P PASS IN MICRONESIA – AND MAKING IT LOOK WAY TOO EASY.

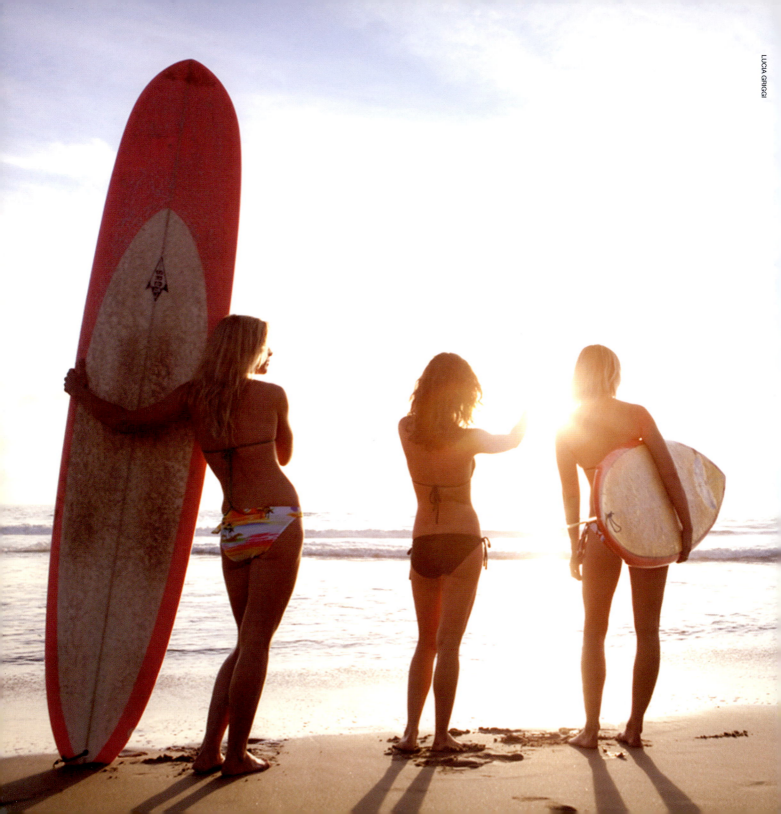

PREPARING FOR TAKEOFF

chapter one

THE OCEAN IS A DANGEROUS PLACE IF YOU DON'T KNOW WHAT YOU'RE DOING, AND IT'S IMPORTANT TO BE WAVE SAVVY. THE KEY TO READING SURF IS IN UNDERSTANDING THE RHYTHM OF NATURE BY ASSESSING SITUATIONS, ANTICIPATING SWELLS, AND LEARNING FROM THOSE WITH MORE EXPERIENCE. THE SOONER YOU DO ALL THREE, THE SOONER YOU'LL BE SPENDING MORE TIME IN THE WATER, AND THE SOONER YOU'LL PROGRESS.

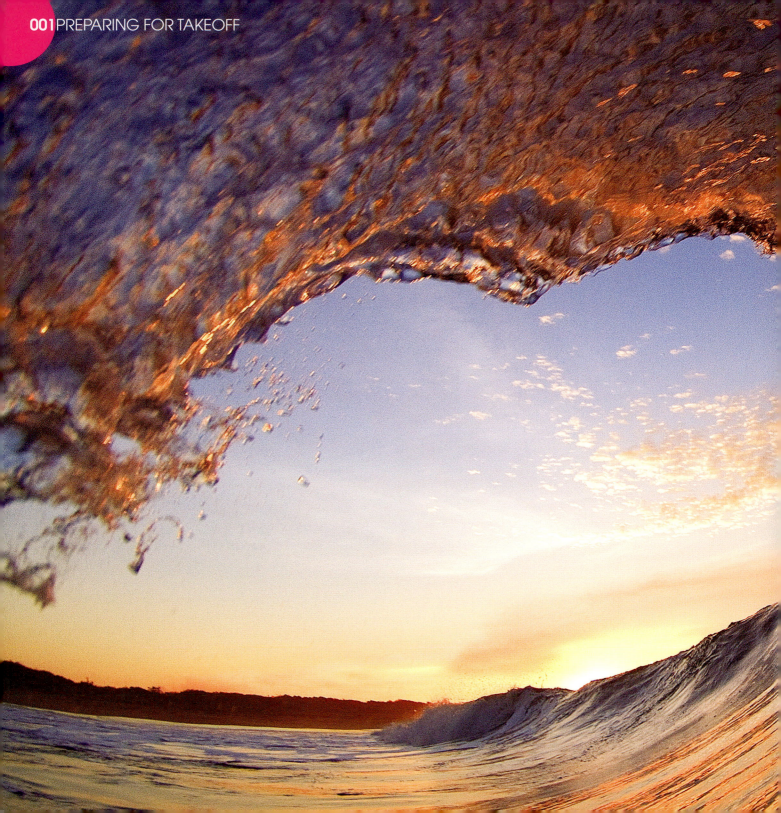

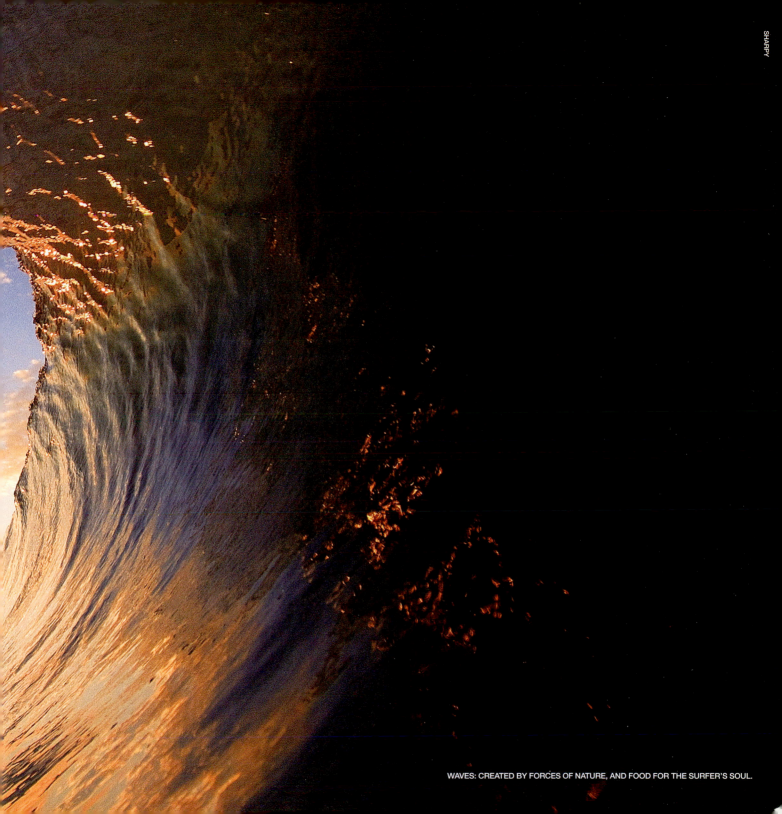

WAVES: CREATED BY FORCES OF NATURE, AND FOOD FOR THE SURFER'S SOUL.

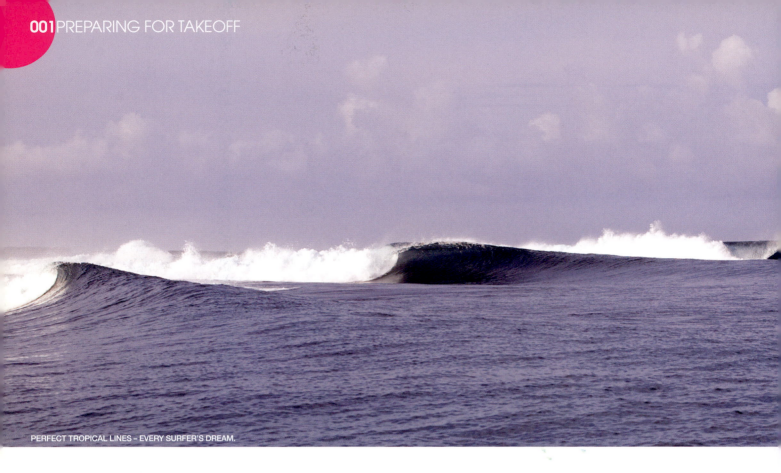

PERFECT TROPICAL LINES – EVERY SURFER'S DREAM.

TYPES OF SWELL

The best types of swell for surfing are groundswells, which are generated many hundreds of miles away by winds revolving around distant low pressure systems. As the swell travels to our beaches it becomes more organised, and classic surfing conditions occur when a solid groundswell combines with an offshore wind – lines of waves can be seen stacked up to the horizon, and the waves themselves are smooth and a joy to ride.

Well organised groundswells are made up of 'trains' of waves, some of which are slightly out of synch with the others. When the crests of two wave trains synchronise, the result is a group of larger waves called a 'set'. Experienced surfers sit and wait for these sets, which arrive at regular intervals, because they're always the biggest and the best waves.

When open-ocean swells move into shallower water they decelerate, 'feel' the seabed, and eventually break as waves. The manner in which waves break depends largely on the configuration of the seabed.

The other main type of swell occurs when a low pressure system passes close to the shore. It brings stormy, windy and wet weather and a different type of swell: windswell. Windswell waves can be just as big as groundswell waves, but tend to be choppy, disorganised, and much closer together... In other words they're rarely as much fun to ride!

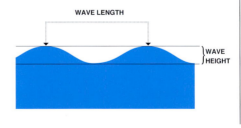

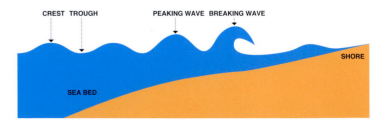

A wave breaks when it reaches a water depth of half its wavelength, the distance between waves.

The land slows down the water at the bottom of the wave, causing the faster upper part, the crest of the wave, to rise and arc, finally crashing down on itself. The crest breaks because it outraces the lower part of the wave and winds up hanging in the air. Gravity draws it back down.

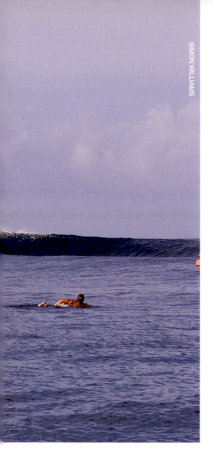

SIMON WILLIAMS

HOW WAVES ARE FORMED

Ocean waves are some of the most complicated phenomena on earth. However, you don't need to become an oceanographer to understand the basics of how waves are formed, and how they break.

Waves come in all shapes and sizes, but they're pretty much all produced the same way: by wind blowing across the ocean and creating swell. (With the exception of tsunamis, which are caused by submarine earthquakes, and tidal waves such as the Severn Bore.)

SWELL PREDICTION

If you live by the coast (or have a boss who'll give you time off whenever you want it!) then you won't have to worry so much about predicting when the next swell's arriving. You can just go to the beach. For the other 99% of us, trying to forecast when the next swell will arrive is an integral part of being a surfer. Especially if you only get to the coast at the weekend. Until recent times surfers were totally dependent on long-range weather forecasts on the telly, and the shipping forecast, but these days you can get an incredibly accurate surf prediction online. www.surfgirlmag.com is a great place to start, and you'll find lots of useful pointers that will tell you when and where the surf will arrive.

Although modern charts and wave prediction sites are pretty idiot proof, it's still useful to know how surf is formed. Learn the basics and then check out the charts for a change: it's quite rewarding!

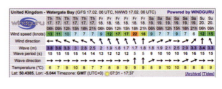

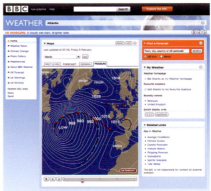

SO, YOU'VE CLICKED ONTO THE SITE AND YOU HAVE WEATHER A CHART IN FRONT OF YOU – WHAT DOES IT ALL MEAN?

• **Isobars are the lines on a weather map.** They represent 'contours' of atmospheric pressure. The important thing to know about isobars is that winds blow roughly parallel to them, and the closer the isobars, the stronger the wind.

• **Low pressure systems (depressions)** are the swirling storm systems that generate most swells as they track across the ocean. The strong winds associated with 'lows' rotate in an anti-clockwise direction.

• **High pressure systems (anti-cyclones)** bring dry sunny weather and light winds, so they usually don't generate much swell. Winds rotate around highs in a clockwise direction.

Three factors determine the size and type of surf generated by a low pressure system: the wind-speed out at sea where the swell is being formed; how long the wind blows for, and the fetch (the distance of open ocean that the wind blows across). Big clean swells are generated by strong winds blowing across a long fetch, hundreds of miles away from where the swell arrives.

As waves travel across long distances they run together and organise themselves, eventually arriving in perfect lines - with regular sets of bigger waves. These sets usually contain four to six waves. Ocean swells generally travel at 20 to 25 mph, so a swell generated by a low in the mid Atlantic will typically take three or four days to arrive on our shores.

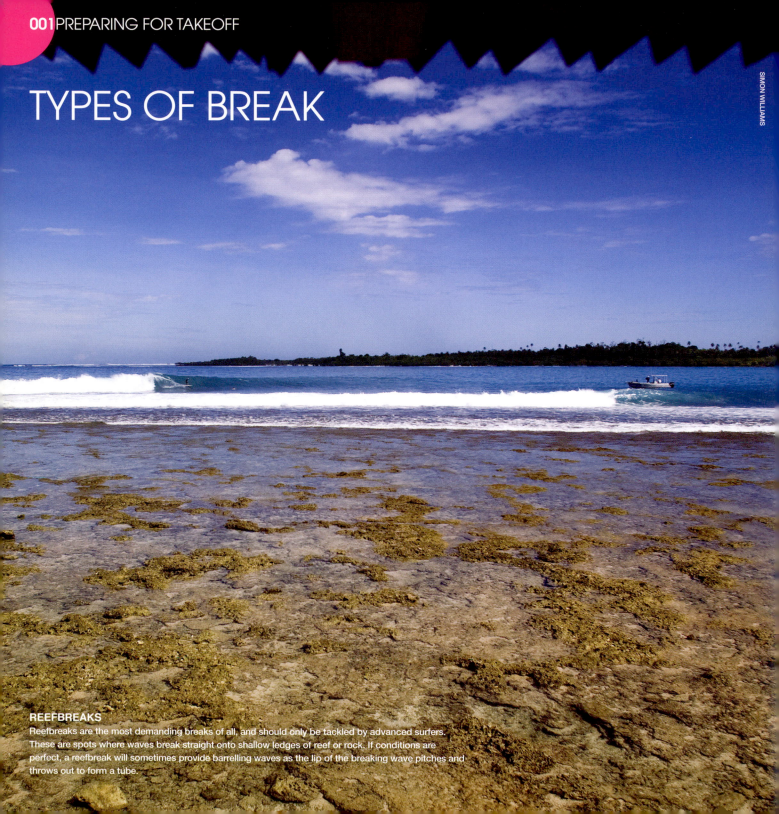

TYPES OF BREAK

SIMON WILLIAMS

REEFBREAKS
Reefbreaks are the most demanding breaks of all, and should only be tackled by advanced surfers. These are spots where waves break straight onto shallow ledges of reef or rock. If conditions are perfect, a reefbreak will sometimes provide barrelling waves as the lip of the breaking wave pitches and throws out to form a tube.

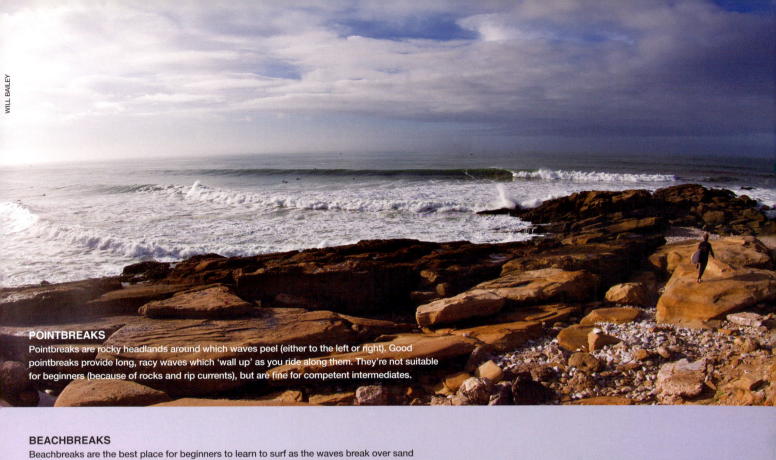

POINTBREAKS

Pointbreaks are rocky headlands around which waves peel (either to the left or right). Good pointbreaks provide long, racy waves which 'wall up' as you ride along them. They're not suitable for beginners (because of rocks and rip currents), but are fine for competent intermediates.

BEACHBREAKS

Beachbreaks are the best place for beginners to learn to surf as the waves break over sand and tend to be slower. The peaks at a beachbreak will move around from one week to another as the sandbars below shift with the currents.

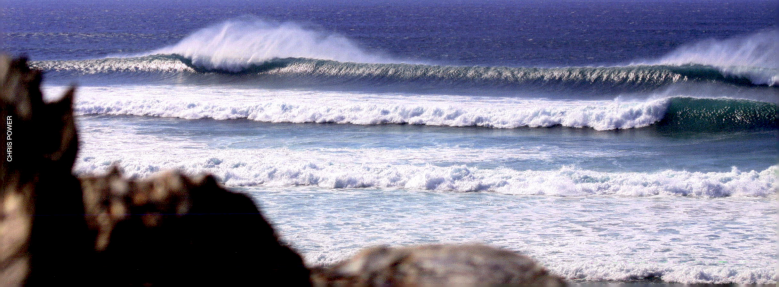

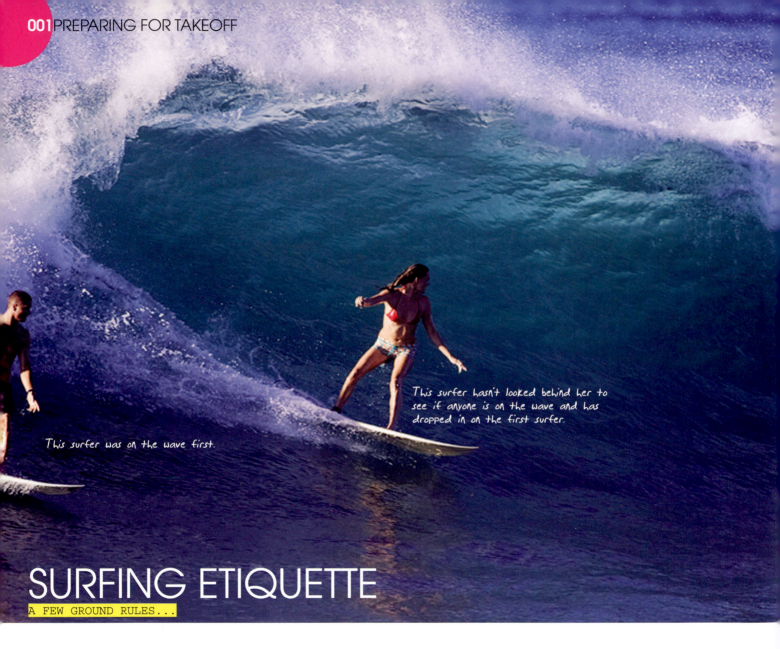

This surfer hasn't looked behind her to see if anyone is on the wave and has dropped in on the first surfer.

This surfer was on the wave first.

SURFING ETIQUETTE
A FEW GROUND RULES...

As well as the basic techniques of surfing that a school will teach you, you'll also come across a number of important ground rules, which apply to all surfers at all times:
• **DON'T surf alone.** It's always safer to surf with mates… And a lot more fun.
• **DON'T surf straight after a meal, or after drinking alcohol.**

• **DON'T bail your board when paddling out through waves if you can possibly help it.** There may be someone right behind you and they won't appreciate getting a board in the face!

Once you've had a few lessons at a surf school, learnt about water safety, and got the right equipment, then it's time to

get out there and learn at your own pace.
   Here are a few things you should do before hitting the water…

• **DO spend a few minutes checking the conditions.** Are there any rips or rocks? How frequent are the sets? Where are the other surfers getting in and out of the water? If there aren't any

other surfers, there's probably a good reason. Maybe the waves are bigger than they look, in which case it could be worth trying a more sheltered spot.
• **DO check your equipment.** Check that your leash is free of nicks or kinks. Wax the deck of your board so it's nice and grippy all over.
• **DO something to warm up your**

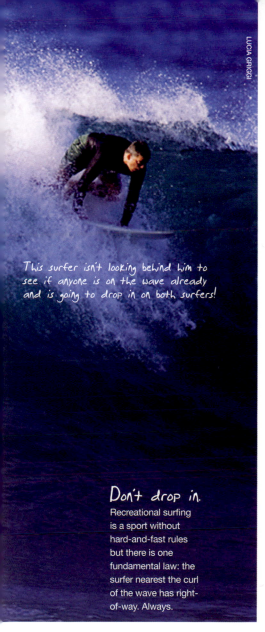

This surfer isn't looking behind him to see if anyone is on the wave already and is going to drop in on both surfers!

Don't drop in.
Recreational surfing is a sport without hard-and-fast rules but there is one fundamental law: the surfer nearest the curl of the wave has right-of-way. Always.

muscles. Cold, stiff muscles and ligaments can easily be wrenched by a wipeout. You can avoid this by warming up thoroughly or spending five minutes jogging (maybe park further from the beach!).
· **DO observe warning flags and restricted-area flags.** These are used for safety purposes by lifeguards at most of the main surfing beaches from late spring to early autumn.

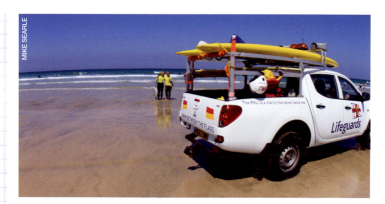

EMERGENCIES

Accidents do happen, it's a fact of life, and whether they're caused by foolishness or plain bad luck makes no difference. At the end of the day the guys who handle tough situations are the guys who know what to do in an emergency.

The following is only intended as a basic guide to emergency action and you should try to get the attention of a lifeguard or call the coastguard as soon as possible. You should also do a course in water safety, rescue skills and resuscitation. The question you should ask yourself is this: if your best friend was in serious trouble, would you know what to do to help?

WATER RESCUE PROCEDURE

If you're on the beach or in the water and you see or hear someone in distress, you may need to perform a water rescue. Here's what to do:

1. Assess the situation. Do NOT risk your own life if you are not sufficiently experienced in the prevailing conditions. Be especially wary of rip currents, rocks and caves. Establish what needs to be done, and what assistance is needed.

2. Send for help. Alert the lifeguards at the nearest lifeguard station, or phone the coastguard. Get assistance from other surfers, especially locals who are likely to be more knowledgeable about the area.

3. If you are completely confident that you can assist the person in trouble without putting your own life at risk, then act quickly. Always use a rescue aid, such as your surfboard or a Peterson tube.

4. The person in trouble may well be distressed or in shock. Talk to them as you approach – try to sound confident, even if you are nervous. When you're about six feet away, pass your board (or rescue aid) to the person. Do not allow them to grab you.

5. Keep the person calm and reassured. If you know help is on its way, it may be best to wait for assistance.

6. If no help is coming, or the situation requires immediate action, place the person on your board and paddle into shore, lying on top of them. Be aware of approaching waves, and keep the patient secure on the board. An unconscious casualty must be brought back to shore as quickly as possible; if they are not breathing, start mouth-to-nose respiration.

7. Once back on the beach, start giving the appropriate aftercare.

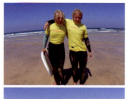

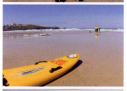

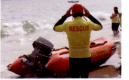

HAZARDS

SURFBOARDS

For beginners, the biggest hazards to watch out for can be surfboards that are out of control. If you see someone else's board hurtling towards you, the best course of action is to duck under the water. Surfboards are very buoyant so if you duck a couple of feet underwater you'll be safe. Cover your head with your arms as you come up to the surface.

ROCKS

If you're surfing a rocky reef or pointbreak then consider wearing a helmet. Try to land feet-first when you wipeout, and never dive off forwards if it's shallow.

WEAVER FISH

Despite their size (six to eight inches long), weaver fish can inflict an excruciatingly painful sting. Weavers are most likely to be encountered at sandy beaches during periods of hot weather, when the fish come into shallow water to spawn. If you get stung (it feels as though you've trodden on a sharp nail), put your foot in a bucket of very hot water (the venom is de-activated by heat) and take a couple of painkillers. Sting relief spray can also help.

JELLYFISH

Jellyfish are the stinging bogeymen of the sea. They come in all shapes and sizes and are found throughout the world's oceans. An encounter with their tentacles can result in everything from a minor irritation through to a full blown venomous sting. Avoid them at all costs and, if stung, seek medical attention immediately.

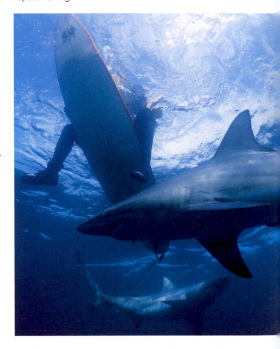
DAVID ALCOCK

SUNBURN

Intense summer sunshine can cause sunburn and increase your risk of getting skin cancer. And being in the water massively increases the effects of the sun. Be smart – use a waterproof sunblock.

TROPICAL DISEASES

In order to avoid potentially life threatening tropical diseases such as malaria and dengue fever, if you are planning a surf trip abroad, the first thing you should do is check which vaccinations are recommended for the areas you will be visiting. Hit the web for info eg www.fitfortravel.nhs.uk/destinations.aspx

CORAL

A major hazard in tropical climes is staph-infested coral. Pack plenty of iodine for coral cuts – even the slightest nick can cause a serious infection – then get medical attention asap.

SHARKS

Considering how many people on the planet spend time in the water, fatal shark attacks are incredibly rare. However, they do occasionally happen and by observing a few basic rules you can drastically reduce your risk.

Stay out of the water at dawn, dusk, and night time – this is when some species of sharks may move inshore to feed.

Do not enter the water if you have open wounds or are bleeding in any way. Sharks can detect blood and body fluids, even in extremely small concentrations.

Avoid murky waters, harbour entrances, channels, steep drop offs, and areas near stream mouths (especially after heavy rains).

Avoid going near people who are fishing or spear fishing.

RIP CURRENTS

Rips are caused by the water pushed towards a beach by the action of waves flowing back out to sea. They can usually be identified from the shore as channels of deeper water (often between sandbars) where the waves aren't breaking: the surface of the water is usually rippled or choppy, and may be discoloured by suspended sand. A strong rip current can quickly drag you out to sea. If you get caught in a rip, don't try to paddle back to shore against the current: paddle across it to wherever the waves are breaking. Rip currents are often only 10 or 20 yards wide, so you can usually escape their clutches quite easily. Never leave your board: it's your life raft.

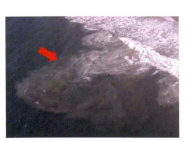

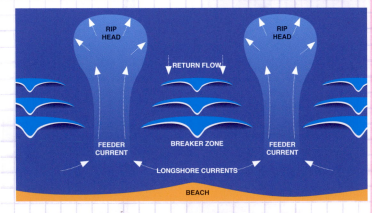

RIP HEAD RIP HEAD
RETURN FLOW
FEEDER CURRENT BREAKER ZONE FEEDER CURRENT
LONGSHORE CURRENTS
BEACH

GETTING STARTED

Surfing can be exhilarating or relaxing, fast or slow, wild or controlled… You can be a mellow longboarder, or a snappy shortboarder and plenty in between because – once you've got it wired – how you ride your board is up to you. But the road to becoming a stand-out ripper at your local break can be a long and challenging one. To give yourself a head start your best bet is to enrol with the pros, and find a decent surf school to guide you through the early days.

SURF SCHOOLS

With an always changing playing field and the specific surf fitness that is required, learning to surf can be a slow and tricky process. Take a look at other sports – tennis, golf, skiing – it's standard to be coached and take lessons if you hope to get anywhere. Surfing's just the same and, through using clear, recognised techniques, lessons can save you hours of struggling on your own. Most schools have a 70% stand up rate in their first lesson and after a week of lessons you will have learned skills that could have taken a year or more to grasp through struggling on your own. Getting the right coaching in the correct environment can dictate whether someone falls in love with surfing, or falls at the first hurdle.

And remember, surf coaching isn't only for novices wanting to try the sport for the first time. Coaching is available for surfers of all abilities, and some of the country's top surfers earn their cash to get away in the winter through working at surf schools in the summer, so they can help you practice your pop, clean up your cutback, or coach you to win a national title!

Most surf schools require clients to be over eight-years-old and over. There's generally no upper age limit, but you need to be able to swim 50 metres in open water. Before choosing a school do some digging and check out their website. Schools that are run professionally and offer good customer service get a good reputation quickly so ask around. Prices will vary depending upon the amount of competition in the area, the time of year and the number of lessons that you sign up for. Remember that cheap isn't necessarily good – you'll find that you get what you pay for in terms of quality and group size.

After your first few lessons, you will always benefit more from signing up for tailored coaching at the correct level for their ability. To improve you need to learn all about:

- Outback surfing
- Ocean awareness
- Surfing etiquette
- Choosing the right equipment for your ability
- Surfing and paddling technique
- Board control
- Safety

Through taking lessons and then clocking up water time to perfect the new techniques, you will learn to surf more quickly and to a much better standard. As your surfing develops you will occasionally feel as though you've reached a plateau in your performance. That's perfectly natural and a great time to get some coaching. Often a few simple words of advice and a demonstration can make a huge difference, and once you're analysed by a professional coach using video feedback, you will realise how to improve and take your surfing to the next level.

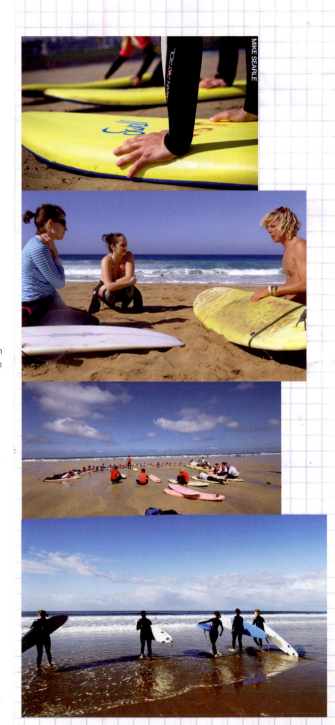

MIKE SEARLE

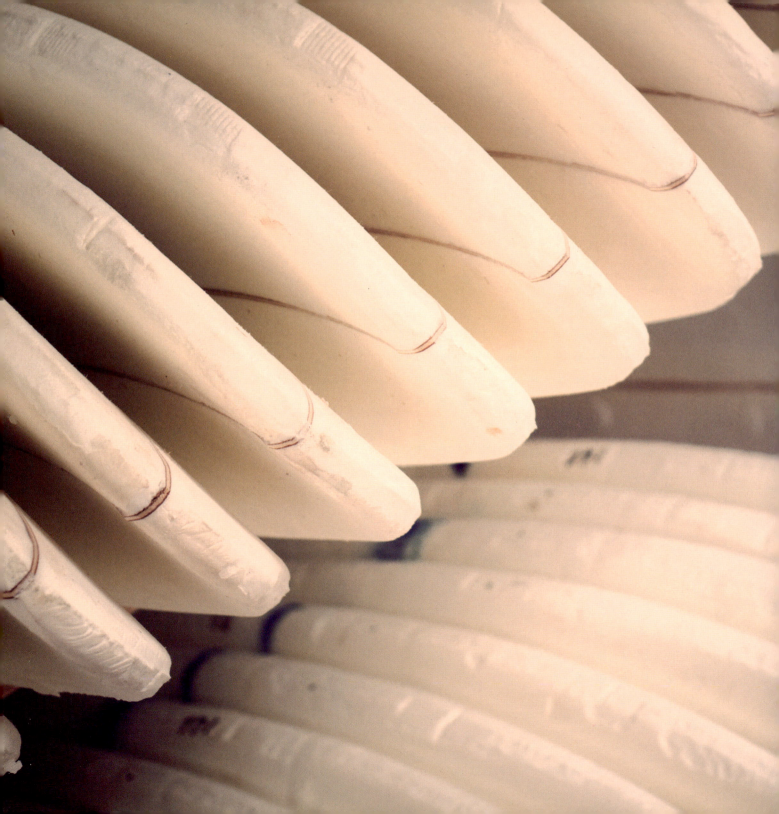

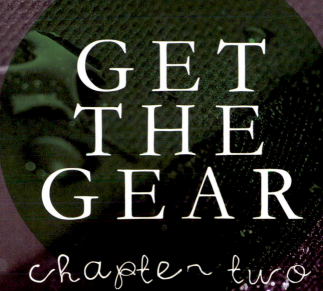

GET
THE
GEAR

chapter two

SURFBOARDS

It's vitally important to pick the right board for your size and ability. This will allow your surfing to develop. Here we take a look at surfboards and how to ensure that you buy your perfect board.

There are three main types of surfboard construction: soft boards, moulded boards, and custom boards, all are available in a range of sizes and shapes.

SOFT SURFBOARDS (or foamies) are made from a semi-rigid plastic foam which is soft and very buoyant. They're very stable and ideal for first-time surfers, and are consequently widely used by surf schools.

MOULDED SURFBOARDS Once you've mastered the basics on a soft board you could move on to a more rigid board which will have much more drive. A moulded board is constructed by joining two moulded-fibreglass halves of the board together, then filling the middle with liquid polyurethane foam which then hardens. Modern moulded boards (brands like NSP and Bic) are harder wearing than custom boards, so they're ideal for novice surfers who've had a few days' tuition at a surf school and want to move on.

CUSTOM SURFBOARDS are made by hand from polyurethane foam blanks which are shaped and then covered with a thin layer of fibreglass. These boards can be made to any shape or design required, and can be sprayed with any colour scheme. They're lightweight, but easily damaged. Suitable for beginners and experts alike, custom boards cost £275-£450.

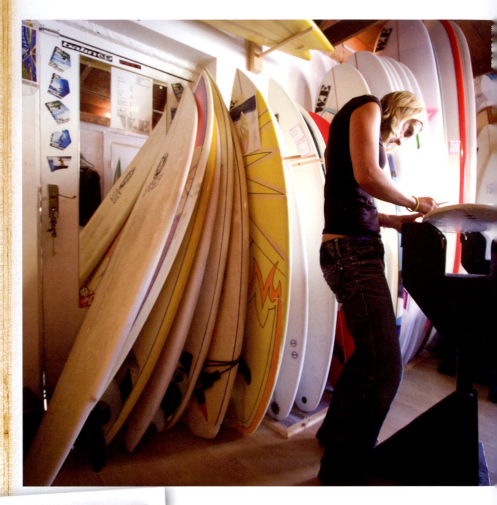

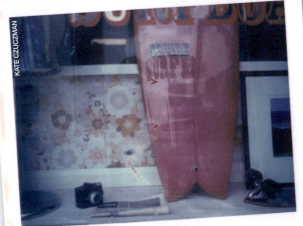

KATE CZUCZMAN

BUYING SECONDHAND

A secondhand board can be a great option – especially if you're hoping to progress quickly and move on to a different board. But check boards over very carefully... A few dents in the deck are nothing to worry about, but delamination (where the outer glass layer has become separated from the foam core) can be a real problem. Dings that have been properly fixed won't affect performance, but avoid snapped boards which have been repaired as these are prone to snap again and the rocker may well be out of line. Again, seek advice from a friend who surfs before buying.

PROGRESSING

As you progress upwards from your lonely struggles in the white water and on to those elusive green faces you're going to want a new board. If you want to be a shortboarder then the fastest way to learn is by gradually reducing your board's length as your skill and strength increases. But remember not to step down too quickly – jumping straight onto a shortboard is just like jumping into a formula one car without taking any lessons. Not only will you not be able to handle the speed and manoeuvrability, but you won't be able to paddle it or catch any waves either. Bad plan! The boards below act as a rough guide through this progression.

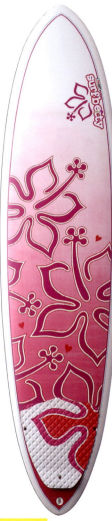

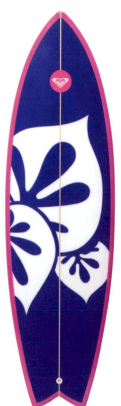

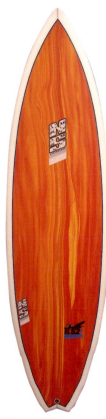

LONGBOARD:

A discipline in its own right, and with as many permutations and combinations as shortboards: from the wafer thin high performance boards to the single fin soul–arch machines. A good choice if you're moving on from a minimal, but you may be limiting yourself in terms of the days that you can make it out back...

MINI–MALS:

The classic first board that has revolutionised the 'learning to surf' experience (no more splashing around on your mate's 5'10"!). Nice and stable with plenty of volume and ideal for getting your confidence in the whitewater, and for taking on your first few unbroken waves. Can be quite cumbersome (and dangerous!) in bigger surf.

FISH:

Fish are shorter than mini–mals, but have plenty of that all important volume. They are nice and easy to catch waves on and will turn and get down the line more quickly than a minimal, but have little rocker and a flat bottom shape so can be hard to handle when it gets bigger.

SHORTBOARD:

Shortboards are the most versatile type of board and can perform quicker turns and more radical manoeuvres than other boards. You can move from a minimal down to a longer shortboard, and you can have high volume shortboards – a clever shaper can squeeze the volume of a 6'6" shortboard into a 6'0" (often a great 'step down' choice).

BUYING A BOARD

Nothing injects a fresh rush of enthusiasm like getting a new board. Here's a few tips to ensure you make the right decision.

Surf shops are a great place to begin your search. It's always good to get the gen from staff who know the boards and the shapers, you can ask as many questions as needs be so that they can help you in your choice. And shop around: even if you think you've definitely found 'that' board, go to a few more shops – it's very easy to fall in love with any shiny new board!

Alternatively, cut out the middle man and go straight to the shaper (just Google surfboard shapers in your local area). Take your old board with you, as a good shaper can glean a lot from looking at this and questioning you about your standard of surfing – be honest, it's not the time to show off! If the shaper has understood your needs properly you should come away with a new board that's going to take your surfing up a level: and it will be one of a kind!

Also lots of shops and shapers have test centres or test shapes so you can borrow them and try before you buy. It's great fun and gives you the opportunity of riding lots of different shapes before parting with your cash. And before you leave the house head to www.surfgirlmag.com, as there's a great board guide to send you off in the right direction.

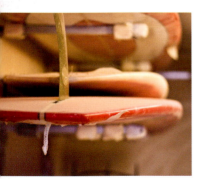

Don't be put off by the jargon. If you can then take someone with you who knows about surfing and has seen you surf, and also check out the shop or shaper's website as they often have lots of in-depth info about their boards so you can buff up before hitting the shops. Then make sure you understand these key elements of surfboard design before you hit the shops and hand over your credit card.

SURFBOARD JARGON...

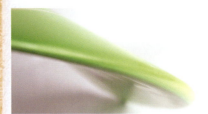

VOLUME. Volume is crucial, and is often overlooked. In simple terms: the more volume you have the better your board floats and the easier it is to paddle and catch waves. But (this is important!) more volume doesn't necessarily mean a longer board – you don't have to stay on a minimal until you've got the upper body strength of Silvana Lima. Lots of shorter boards nowadays have as much volume as boards half a foot longer, so you get all the benefits of 'less board' without the arm ache and frustration.

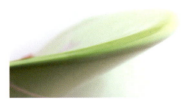

ROCKER. This is how much bend is in your board (a board with a lot of rocker looking more like a banana!). Having more rocker enables you to get your board into more critical sections of the wave, but too much also means that your board is 'pushing more water' when you're paddling it, or if the waves are sloppy (lots of boards shaped overseas have too much rocker for typical UK waves). If you aren't quite at the 'ripping' stage yet, then steer clear of anything too radical in the rocker department.

RAILS. Rails (the edges of the board) come in all shapes and sizes and have a lot more to them than you would credit when you're looking down a row of gleaming new boards. In simple terms

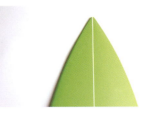

you have 'soft rails' and 'hard rails'. On a soft rail the edge of the board has an even, semi circular contour, whereas on a hard rail the curve is nearer the bottom of the board. Hard rails make a board more responsive but less forgiving, whereas soft rails give you a bit more leeway. All boards have hard rails towards the tail which become softer as you move up the board, but there are an infinite number of permutations...

TAIL. A few years ago tail types were pretty clear-cut, but the waters have become more muddied in recent times and many modern tails are a mixture. The most widely used and versatile tail is a squash tail (imagine your board with a totally square tail, and then just round the edges off neatly!). This type of tail is wide and quite forgiving and is good for most types of surf. For bigger days and more critical waves a pin tail has less area and allows the water a smooth exit from the board so is the choice of big wave riders and tube-hounds. The rounded pin is the more common 'in between' option offering speed and manoeuvrability. A swallow tail is the easiest tail to spot as, well, it looks like a swallow's tail! It shares similar characteristics with the other main tail types: wider for stability, but with similar 'hold' on the wave to a pintail.

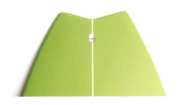

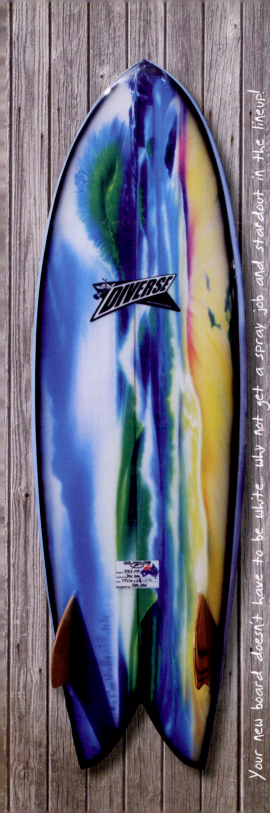

Your new board doesn't have to be white... why not get a spray job and stand out in the lineup!

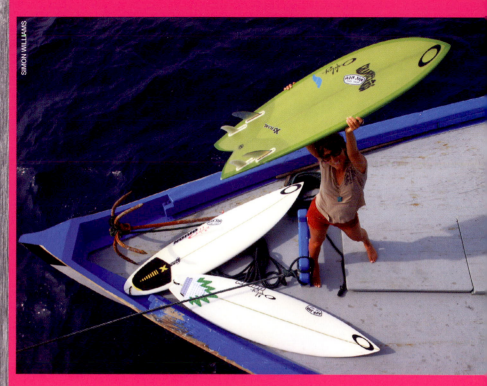

SIMON WILLIAMS

ASK THE EXPERTS

HOW MUCH SHOULD I PAY?

The most important thing about getting a board is choosing the right one for where you're at with your surfing, and for the style of surfing that you're in to. So you don't need to spend lots of money on an expensive board 'cos you like the spray, but don't spend too little beacuse it's cheap on eBay because, well, it was only £50!

Work out what your perfect stick is, set yourself a price limit, and go find it. It will be out there.

DO GIRLS NEED DIFFERENT BOARDS TO BOYS?

There isn't really a black and white answer here, as Phil Bridges at Tiki Surfboards explains, "It's easy to generalise when suggesting

boards to girls and offer the same board but perhaps a bit smaller or thinner. In reality it's more complex than that: girls have smaller feet, are lighter and have less powerful shoulders (but more natural grace!). If you offer a standard off-the-peg model but smaller to girls, then it may be hard to paddle.

For a guy finding it hard to paddle a shorter board you might suggest a wider template, like a fish, but for girls these wide tailed boards are hard to turn without being able to apply pressure directly on the rail. Tiki did a board test day with SurfGirl a couple of years ago and by far the most appropriate board turned out to be a small Magic Carpet style board. The combination of wide front section for paddling and narrow round pin tail which could easily be 'leant' into a turn proved to be a winner."

SO HOW DO I FIND MY 'MAGIC BOARD'?

We're all different, as Trevor Clayton from Down The Line Surf Shop says, "Some surfers like super-rockered wafers, some flatter, thicker boards. There's no right or wrong – just what works for you. Try everything once, use any test centres you can, never write off any advice, and talk to shapers and salesmen. You'll be glad you did." So, be open minded, do try different boards (an awareness of how different shapes perform will improve your overall surfing too), and get to know what works for you.

Once you've found your magic board then get to know it well and don't chop and change. Work on building a good relationship with your shaper or shop salesman and it could be the start of a beautiful partnership!

WETSUITS

Wetsuits these days are better made, lighter, and stretchier than ever before and you get a lot more bang for your buck than a few years ago. Here's some tips on deciding which wetsuit is for you.

Shopping for a wetsuit isn't like shopping for a pair of jeans where your biggest concern may be "how does my butt look in these?!" There's a whole world of decisions to make before you decide which is the right wetsuit for you (and no, how your butt looks doesn't come into it!).

Heading into your local surf shop can be a daunting experience – as can shelling out that much cash – so ask the right questions and know what you're looking for before you hand over your credit card. Run through the wetsuit features and know what they mean so you're not blinded by the shop assistant's jargon. Know the difference between flatlock and blindstitched.

When you've got the suit on check for baggy areas in the back, under the arms and on the back of your knees. There shouldn't be much slack material here. Or around your breasts, make sure it all fits snugly. Make sure the neck, wrist and ankle seals are ok. They should feel tight, but not so tight that your hands turn blue.

Try out a few entry systems, and check out the difference between chest zip, back zip and short zip before you buy. Chest zips are great as no water can get in through the zip when you duck-dive or are sat on your board – but they can be quite tricky to get into!

A common problem area is the neck. Too tight and it can rub, and too loose and it will flush through. Choose an entry system that's tight but doesn't throttle you, and one that allows for adjustment. Then stretch in your suit – you may feel a bit of a plum but do some star jumps and squats: you need to find a suit that isn't baggy and has the best range of movement.

Shop assistants are there to help you and they're usually genned up on which are the best suits for your budget – so use their knowledge. And try on as many suits as you need to. It can be sweaty and generally quite uncomfortable after your fifth suit: but you have to go through it! Put plastic bags on your feet, this helps to ease them in and out of your suit, and go to a few different shops and try on suits in your budget from as many companies as you can.

Don't skimp! You get what you pay for, and the more you spend the more features your suit will have. If you can't afford the top-of-the-range suits then prioritise flexible neoprene, an entry system that suits you, and good seams – ideally liquid sealed. (And maybe put that bikini fund towards your wettie instead!)

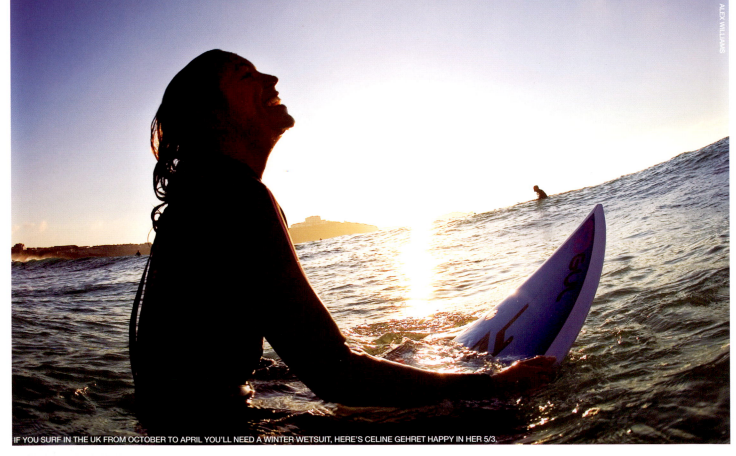

ALEX WILLIAMS

IF YOU SURF IN THE UK FROM OCTOBER TO APRIL YOU'LL NEED A WINTER WETSUIT, HERE'S CELINE GEHRET HAPPY IN HER 5/3.

WETSUIT JARGON

Hyperstretchliquidsealedwhat? It's a confusing old world out there in wetsuit land, so here's a rundown of some of the key terms to get your head round.

3/2 Depending on the individual design, a 3/2 suit generally has three millimetres of neoprene on the torso (where warmth is paramount) and two millimetres elsewhere (for more flexibility). You'll need a 3/2 for the summer months and a 5/3 for the winter.

GLUED AND BLINDSTITCHED edges are glued together then stitched – stitching pierces only the inside layer of the neoprene so the join is nearly watertight.

FLATLOCK STITCHING summer suits are often flatlocked. Two overlapping edges of material are stitched together and the finished seam lies flat inside and outside.

OVERLOCK STITCHING the most basic form for budget suits. It leaves seams on the inside which is less watertight and less comfortable.

LIQUID SEAL SEAMS (LQS) a trail of latex-based glue put onto seams to create a waterproof and flexible seal. Stitching creates holes, so sealing is a good idea.

CRITICALLY TAPED tape glued to maximum stress seams like shoulders to keep them extra-strong. A suit can also be fully taped.

SMOOTH SKIN/GLIDE SKIN slippy, thin neoprene generally used on neck seals. Doesn't rub and goes on and off easily. Often used on barrier/back seals as well.

SIMULATED MESH SKIN, DURASKIN AND SIMILAR outer covering on chest and back panels to repel water, prevent wind-chill and increase durability.

BARRIER SYSTEM, BATWING systems of flaps inside the back which arrange to give you the least amount of drip and flush possible. A good idea.

3/4 ZIP the most common form of zip which does up the back.

CHEST ZIP a panel pulls over your head from your back and you zip it up across the chest. A more flexible construction which leaves your back and shoulders free to move and prevents water from getting in through the zip.

THERMOSPAN / FIREWALL / CORE / POLYPRO PANELS fancy names for a lovely layer of insulating material which draws water away from the body. Usually on chest and maybe back panels where your vital organs need the protection.

WRIST AND ANKLE SEALS liquid seam sealant is often put around the inside of wrists and ankles so that they will seal tight onto the smooth neoprene of your gloves and boots.

HYDROPHOBIC literally: water phobic. Repels water.

SINGLE LINED single lined neoprene has only one layer of fabric, double has one on each side. Single is more flexible, double is more durable and warmer.

For more info on buying wetsuits go to www.surfgirlmag.com

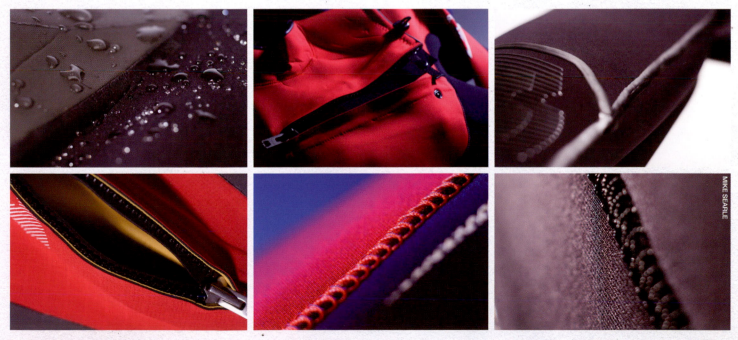

MIKE SEARLE

ACCESSORIES

Once you're well equipped with your board and wettie, make sure you've done your research and invested in the following accessories...

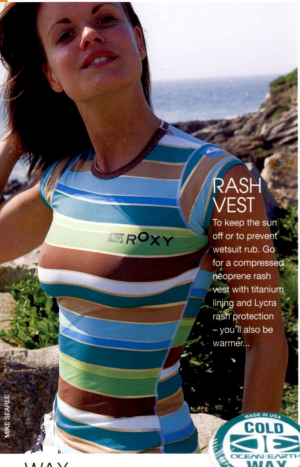

MIKE SEARLE

DECK GRIP

A deck grip sits at the back of the board and provides good solid traction for your back foot. There are various options, some with 'tail kicks' or foot arch support: before you buy one put it on the ground, step on, and see how it feels.

LEASH

Your leash stops you having to endlessly swim back to shore to get your board after you've wiped out. It is a stretchy urethane cord fixed to the tail of the surfboard and attached to your ankle by a velcro wraparound strap. When choosing a leash look at your board's length and choose a leash targeted to that size – longer board equals longer leash.

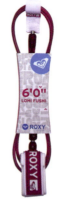

RASH VEST

To keep the sun off or to prevent wetsuit rub. Go for a compressed neoprene rash vest with titanium lining and Lycra rash protection – you'll also be warmer...

NOSEGUARD

If you've decided to shortboard then you're going to want a noseguard – a rubber mould to glue on the tip of your board. A noseguard prevents injuries when you wipeout. Injuries are pretty rare, but when they do occur they tend to be as a result of collision between you and either the nose or fins of your board. Better safe than sorry!

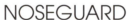

WAX

You need to apply a liberal layer of 'base' wax on a new board to give you grip, and then a light coat of wax each time you surf. You should apply it mostly where your feet are going to be positioned, but it's good to have a bit all over for added grip, and on the rails where you push up with your hands.

WETSUIT BAGS

There are a wide variety of wetsuit bags, from backpacks with wet and dry pockets, through to changing mats that transform into bags which also protect your suit when you're getting in and out of it.

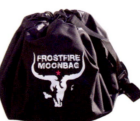

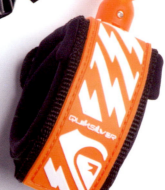

BOARD BAGS

Made from high density foam padding, with a tough fabric exterior, a boardbag is essential if you live anywhere other than next to the beach! Your boards aren't cheap, so invest in a decent board bag and protect them at home or abroad.

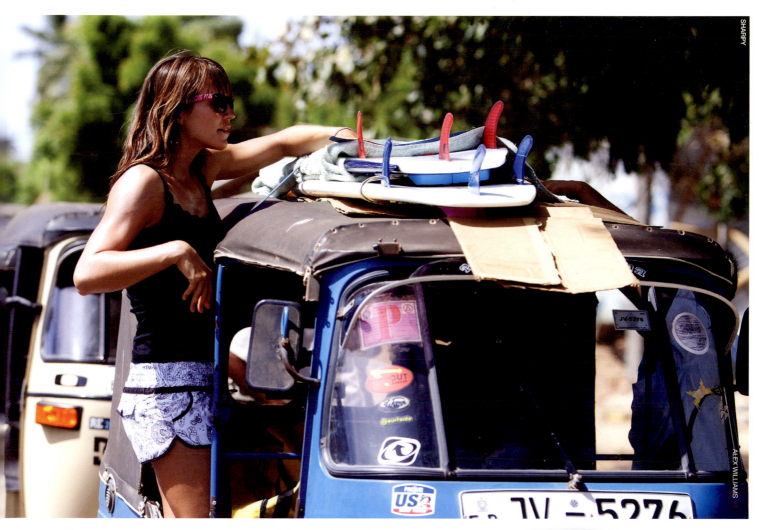

SHARPY

ALEX WILLIAMS

EQUIPMENT TIPS

How to strap your boards on the roof... (Don't leave it to the boys, muck in with the board-loading and you'll get to the waves faster!)

1. Load the boards up biggest first, nose at the front and deck down, with an equal amount of board on each side of the roofracks. Snuggle the tails close together in between the fins of the board below. The stack should end up with an equal amount of tail and nose overhang.

2. Put towels between boards if they are not in bags (wax on the bottom and extra grindage will occur otherwise).

3. Lay the straps (we're using two) over the top of the stacks, one over the front roof bar and one over the back. Thread them through any boardbag straps available and/or between the fins.

4. If there's no roofrack then open all the doors and fasten the straps on the inside of the car. Tighten straps (hard!) and close door. NB: Try not to do this in front of the hire car depot. They don't like it.

5. If you've got a roofrack, loop the strap over the bar on the other side of the car, feed it back over, into the buckle and pull hard, then tie off with a few half hitches

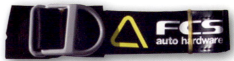

(or a granny knot!).

6. If you've got straps with D-rings (the ultimate) or the more usual buckle system, make sure you've threaded the strap through untwisted. These types of straps will pull tighter and are more securely.

7. Grab the stack and try to pull it off. If it moves at all, tighten the straps.

8. Keep checking those boards as you belt it down the motorway!

KEEPING YOUR GEAR SAFE AND SECURE

Losing expensive surf gear to pesky thieves isn't a pleasant experience and can ruin your day out, or your holiday. Here are a few tips for securing your gear at home and abroad.

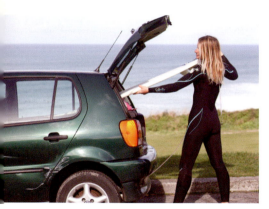

IN THE CAR

• Park in as highly-visible a spot as possible.

• Your car is a shop window for thieves. Lock it, alarm it if possible, and never leave the keys on or near it!

• Don't leave valuables on show. If there's nothing of value in the glove box (and there really shouldn't be!) leave it open so thieves can see there's no point.

• Keep your keys safe. Many beaches offer a key-minding service, but your best bet is a waterproof wallet like the Ocean & Earth water wallet, or the Aquapac Keymaster which comes with a neck cord and will float if dropped. Space for keys, cash, asthma inhalers… It's guaranteed 100% waterproof to 150 feet and is dust and sand-proof as well.

• If you don't have a fancy electronic key, just string it around your neck. Wetsuit and leash pockets are an option too, but slightly less secure. There are some products on the market which will lock your key away behind a combination, but as these are still on the car they can void your insurance, so check first.

ABROAD

Keep all your gear with you and don't leave it on balconies or patios. Even if the locals are cool, fellow travellers might not be. If you're stashing things, hide them in different places so you're less likely to lose it all. This applies to hiding money too – get a good security belt: one with wire sewn into the strap so it can't be cut off you.

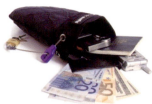

The PacSafe TravelSafe 100 is a favourite travel companion – a compact, lightweight security pouch which is ideally sized and is made of a tightly-woven stainless steel mesh so it can't be cut open, and a strong steel coil you can use like a bike lock. This can live in your car home or abroad and also be used in hostels, on the beach and so on. Secure it to something solid then drop a towel over it so no-one's any the wiser.

If you fall asleep on the plane/bus/train, you're at risk. Don't leave bags in luggage racks any distance from your seat. Put them above your head or under the seat and squash your valuables up close to you so they're not easily moved.

Don't leave anything of value in a hire car – they're often targets. Buy a local sticker to make you look less like a tourist and don't leave tons of maps on the dashboard. Lock your doors while you're driving around.

If you're heading out for a long trip, make an inventory of all your gear, take a photo and mark everything with UV pen. Note serial numbers and make copies of all your important documents and credit cards – if you lose your passport having a copy will really help with red tape. Leave some copies with family or friends at home. Consider having a small USB key with all your vital details encrypted on it.

Get good travel insurance that insures your kit too (check that small print!). Try www.Surfboard-Tracker.com, 'DNA for your board', which will get your board logged worldwide via a little implanted chip.

A tatty old boardbag is less of a target, so think about patching the old girl up and saving yourself some money as well. It's the same for other gear – don't take the best new-season clothes and equipment to poor countries, then you don't have to worry about it.

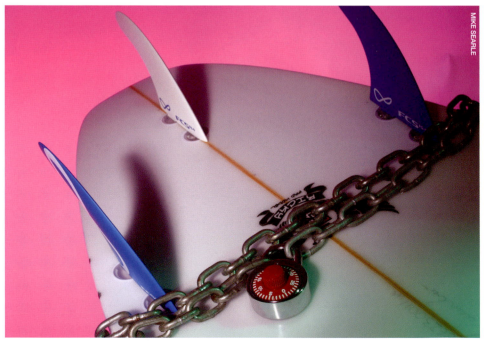

MIKE SEARLE

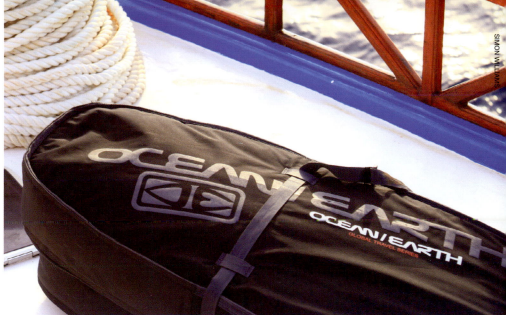

CRUNCH TIME

Patching up your wetsuit and plugging up the holes in your board – it's not a permanent solution, or even the prettiest, but in the spirit of saving money and reducing your consumption of petrochemical by-products, it's the way to go.

BOARD CARE – PROTECTION

Most dings happen on land, a fact that is all too apparent to most of us. So protect your board while in the house, the car or (lucky you) when heading abroad.

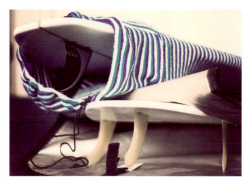

BOARDBAGS

• Choose one for your type of board as well as its length – if you have a fat fish you'll need a retro-style bag for example.
• Boardsocks are a simple and cost-effective way to protect your board.
• Boardbags are made from 1mm to 6mm foam with polyester outside layers and often a UV-reflecting silver material called 'tarpee' which prevents your board heating up in sunlight. Most have plenty of space and often vents to allow air in. There's usually a pocket for fins and wax, a padded shoulder strap and a carry handle.

DINGS

EMERGENCY: Remove all wax, sand and dirt from the area then dry it off.

Plug the hole with a bit of wax then slap a sticker over the top. This should keep the water out for a session or so, but is only a last-ditch measure.

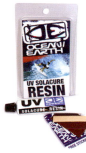

QUICK FIX: The most basic kind of ding repair kit is a simple tube of premixed resin like the Ocean & Earth Solacure kit. Remove all wax, sand and dirt from the area then dry it off. Mix a ball of Solacure together and then plug the hole with it. Dry it out in sunlight and you can be back in the water in a couple of hours.

DIY: Buy a proper ding repair kit – a good investment. It should contain everything you need for a decent ding

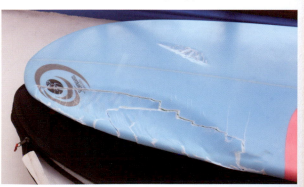

repair session: resin especially formulated for repair use, catalyst (or hardener), a flat spatula, spare foam and fibreglass matting, sandpaper, gloves and mixing cups. Clean and sand as before, then mix the resin and hardener according to the instructions given and fill the hole. Chop up small bits of matting to fill larger holes. Let it all dry thoroughly then you can sand it down again.

The kits come with a full set of instructions, but if you want to get good at fixing dings, the Ding Repair Scriptures is widely recognised as the bible of ding repair.

PRO: Start off fixing small dings and work your way up. When you find you need to use an angle-grinder or be there for a year sanding, it's time to call in the pros (unless you have an angle grinder…).

PATCH IT UP

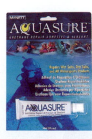

Your suit might last an extra season if you look after it and fix any tears that may appear. Get some strong thread and a fairly thick needle and some wetsuit glue from your local surf shop – Aquasure is the industry standard! Make sure your wetty is clean and dry, then stitch up any seams that have come undone. Follow up with a good blob of glue. If you're gluing boots, rub some sand into the half-dry repair so that you don't end up with a slick sole!

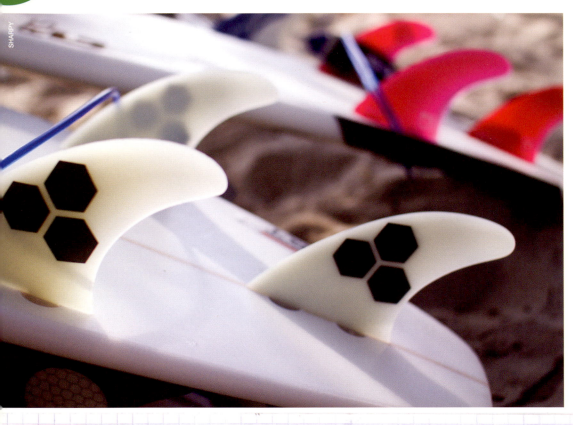

FINS

You know they're there, but beyond trying to work out how to wrap your leash around them in under five minutes and not ride them into the sand, you don't really think about them. What are fins for anyway, and how do they work?

Basically, fins stabilise your board and stop it skipping about like a skimboard, as well as creating drive (forward movement) to allow you to turn. Fin selection is always a trade-off and it's worth playing around with your fins to balance out stability and manoeuvrability.

Until the late '90s, most boards were made with fixed fins which were glassed on, and fin design was in its infancy. Now you can choose from 75 designs of removable fin in the latest FCS brochure alone! Removable fins allow you to change how your board surfs to suit the waves or your riding, as well as allowing you to remove them for travel and reduce the chance of damage. There are a few different fin systems, for example FCS, Future and Lok Box.

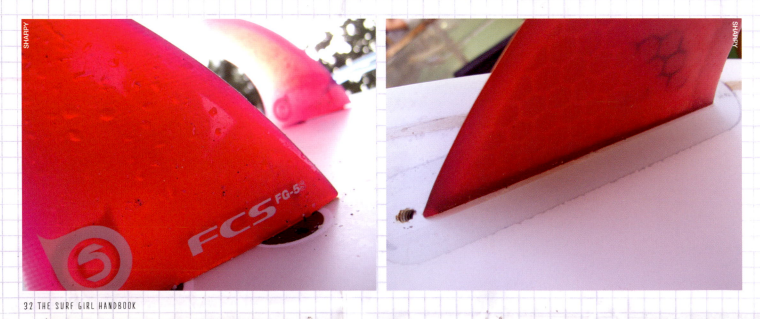

ANATOMY OF A FIN

DEPTH
How long the fin is from the tip to where it joins the board. The longer the fin, the more it will hold in the water. The trade-off is ease of turning – smaller fins will allow the board to manoeuvre more easily.

BASE
The length of the bottom of the fin where it meets the board. More base gives more drive (acceleration) as there is more area to push against the water. Less base means the board will turn more tightly.

FIN PLUGS
These tabs of plastic slot into the fin boxes on the board and screw in with little screws called grub screws which require a special hex key. Keep spares of keys and screws, and don't screw your fins in too hard or you'll strip the screws. Fin systems other than FCS may use slightly different setups.

RAKE OR SWEEP
The curve of the fin. A smaller angle gives better drive, a larger rake gives more manoeuvrability.

FLEX
This is the amount of side to side movement – grab a fin and give it a wiggle. Beginner's boards tend to have flexier fins, these are more forgiving and give more drive but slower turns.

FOIL
The 'bulge' of the fin. Foil determines how much lift and drag a fin has and works in a similar way to aeroplane wings. If you're on a thruster, the middle fin will have foil on both sides while the outer two fins will most likely have foil on the outside and a flat inside. More water flows over the curved outside edge of the fin (the foiled bit) than the flat inside edge and this difference in pressure and speed creates suction or lift, which holds the board into the wave. The board feels faster and responds better through turns.

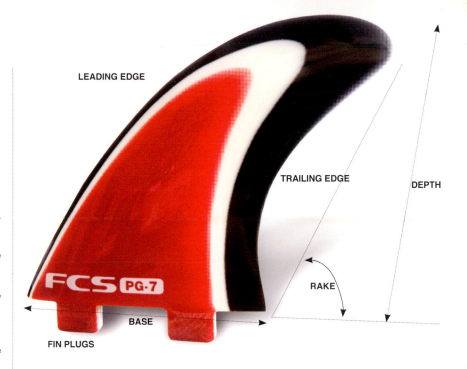

LEADING EDGE

TRAILING EDGE

DEPTH

RAKE

FCS PG-7

BASE

FIN PLUGS

So how do you put this into practice? Think of your surfing and your board, and if there's something you'd like to change, testing a new set of fins might just help. So, if for example your board loses it on turns (slips out), try bigger fins to dig into the wall. If it turns slowly (you have to nurse or force it through turns), try smaller fins to loosen the board up. If you're a heavier person, try bigger fins – more surface area will provide more hold.

On some boards (commonly long and retro boards), you can move the fins backwards and forwards in the box. If you move them forwards, you'll get more response and if backwards, you'll see more hold and drive. If you take the centre fin of a thruster out altogether, you can see how it feels to ride a twinny – fast, loose and skatey.

This all depends on how you surf (you may be more heavy on one foot, for example), so it's important to try variations until you're happy. While it won't make much difference while you're a beginner, once you can traverse the open wave face, knowing a bit about fins will mean you can extend the life of a board or transform it altogether. Packs of fins in shops and online will state exactly what they're designed to do for a board, as well as often being rated for the surfer's weight, so do a bit of research and presto, the perfect fins.

MAKING YOUR EQUIPMENT LAST LONGER

• Keep your board in a bag and somewhere out of harm's way.
• Always wash your wetsuit, hang and dry out of direct sunlight.
• As soon as a ding or tear appears, get it fixed before it goes beyond repair.
• The most cost-effective solution might well be to get it done by a pro – don't waste money and time if you aren't confident you can sort it yourself.
• Regularly re-wax your board to keep the traction fresh – you can check for dings hidden under the wax at the same time.

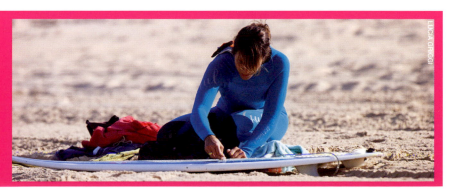

Kassia Meador

The ability to express yourself in the water is an essential part of surfing and Californian Roxy longboarder Kassia Meador sums up the grace and style of longboarding today. Kassia epitomises that 'Malibu' vibe; her graceful style, the boards she rides and her quirky photography all have that rich retro feel.

Hi Kassia, what did you learn to surf on?
I learned to surf on a 7'6" blaster that my dad had.

What keeps you riding Retro shapes?
I like things that are a bit old fashioned, but with a modern twist. I love the glide and trim of a log, the lines you can take on a fish, and the speed and connection I feel to the wave when I'm surfing an alaia. I guess I just love the way different shapes bring you to a different place on a wave, and how each is unique in its own way. Surfing is about freedom and creativity. I have the most fun and get the most out of it when I ride what I want, when I want, and when I keep my mind open to trying new boards.

What boards are you riding at the moment?
The boards I ride most often are my log, my alaia and one of my fishes – either my twinny or my quad. Sometimes I'll ride a tri fin, but a smaller one with a bit more volume. I also love body surfing and getting my hand plane out.

What's your favourite board and why?
I love them all equally in a different way... It just depends what the waves are like when I go out. Sometimes I'll walk two down to the beach and switch over because I am a tripper and just can't get enough variety! I mean it's the spice of life, right?

Interview by Izzy Keene

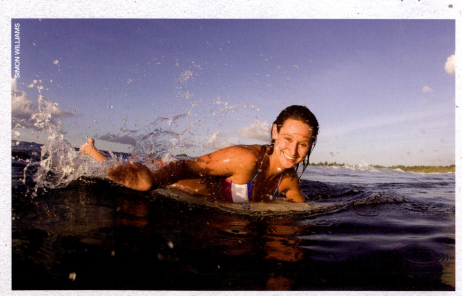

SIMON WILLIAMS

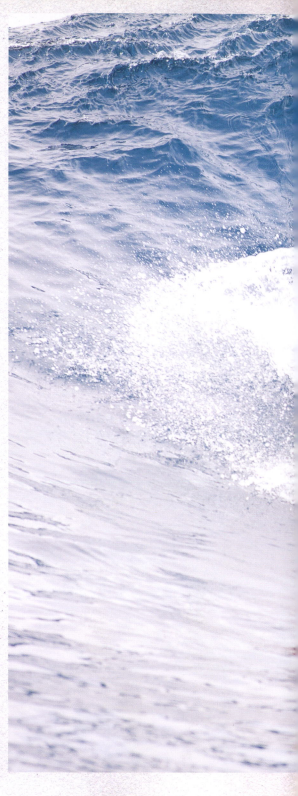

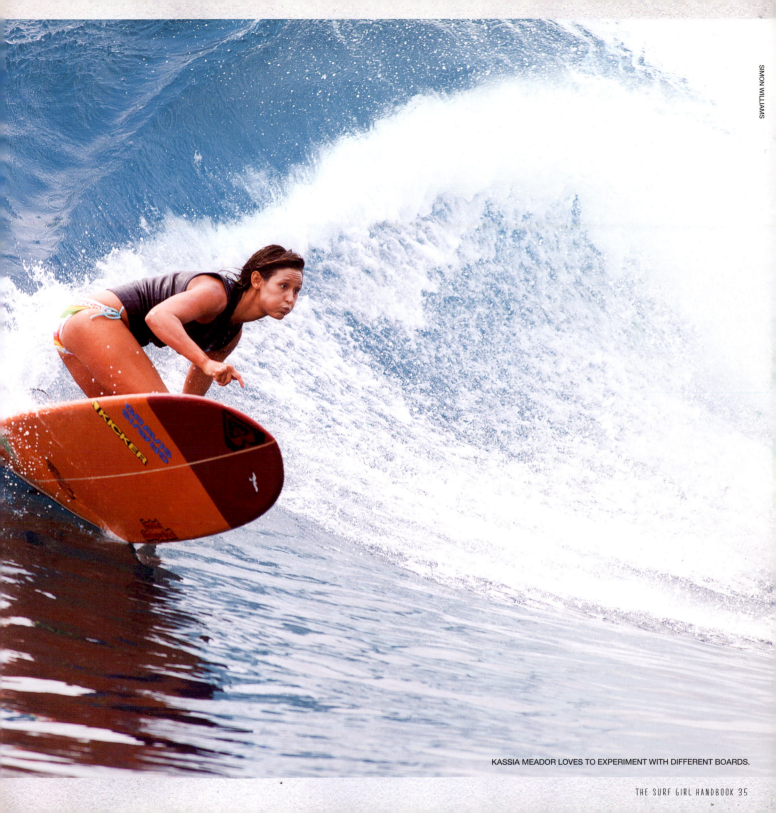

KASSIA MEADOR LOVES TO EXPERIMENT WITH DIFFERENT BOARDS.

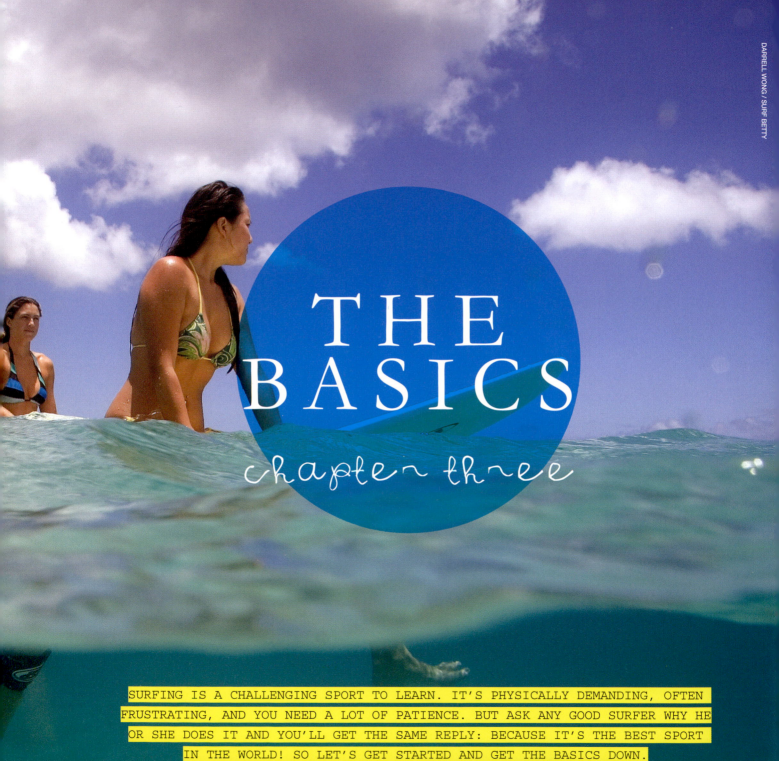

THE BASICS

chapter three

SURFING IS A CHALLENGING SPORT TO LEARN. IT'S PHYSICALLY DEMANDING, OFTEN FRUSTRATING, AND YOU NEED A LOT OF PATIENCE. BUT ASK ANY GOOD SURFER WHY HE OR SHE DOES IT AND YOU'LL GET THE SAME REPLY: BECAUSE IT'S THE BEST SPORT IN THE WORLD! SO LET'S GET STARTED AND GET THE BASICS DOWN.

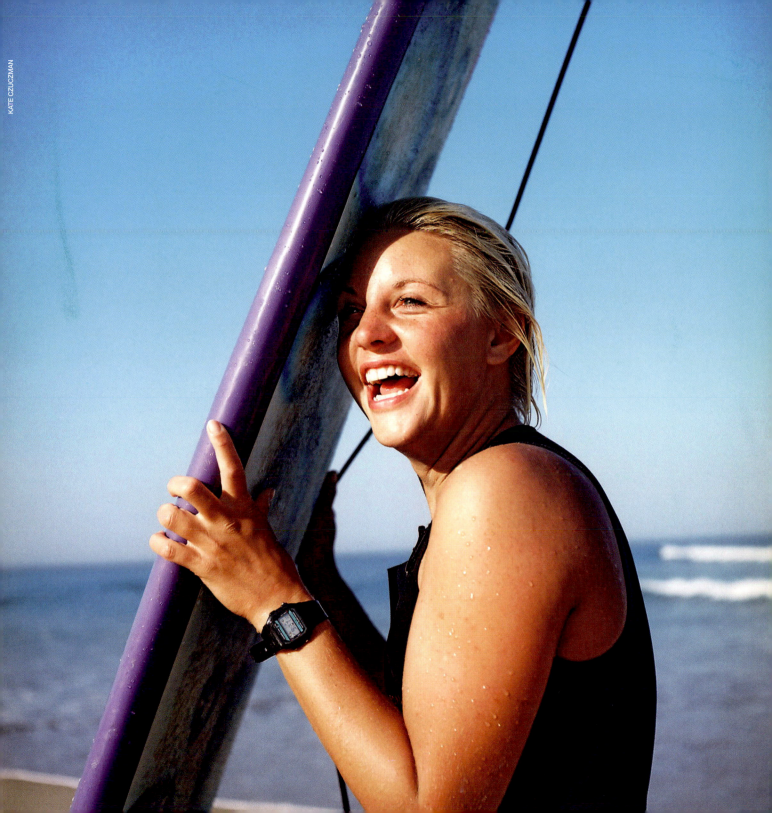

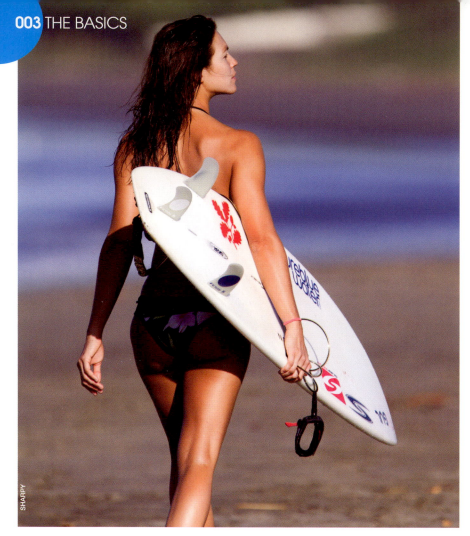

SHARPY

CARRYING YOUR BOARD

To begin with it may sound pretty basic but once you've got your own board, you don't want to destroy it by dragging it along the beach – or worse still, injure somebody.

You need to learn how to carry it under your arm. There are three ways to do this;

• The first is to put the fin in towards your body, although this can be difficult if you don't have the arm length.

• The second way is to put the fin in front of you turned inwards so that you can see it and can avoid hitting anyone with it. Then the curve of the board is against your body so it is easier to get your arm around it. Remember that if you are carrying your board with the deck against your body you will get wax all over you. This doesn't matter if you're in your wetsuit but if you're walking to the beach with your new Roxy top on it will get gunked up.

• If you have a longer board, say 7" and upwards, it's best to partner up with someone with a similar length board. You can carry both the tails of the board and your partner can carry both the noses.

Make sure that you have the leash wrapped around the tail of the board or you carry it in the same hand as the one that you are carrying the board with. This will save you tripping over it. Remember, carrying your board is a bit like carrying a ladder, if you turn around quickly the board will turn in a big circle, so be careful not to hit anyone with the fin.

WALKING OUT

Right it's now time to hit the water. Remember, it's best to go out in small, clean waves at a sandy beach while you're learning. First of all walk out to waist depth water, making sure your surfboard is pointing straight out to sea. Hold your board to one side. You don't want your surfboard between you and the wave, as the board can hit you.

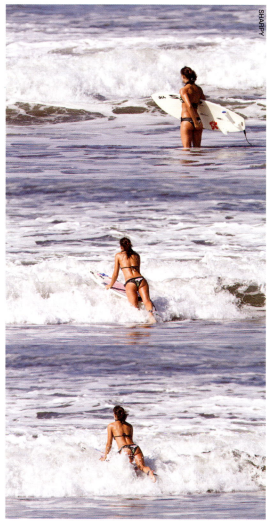

SHARPY

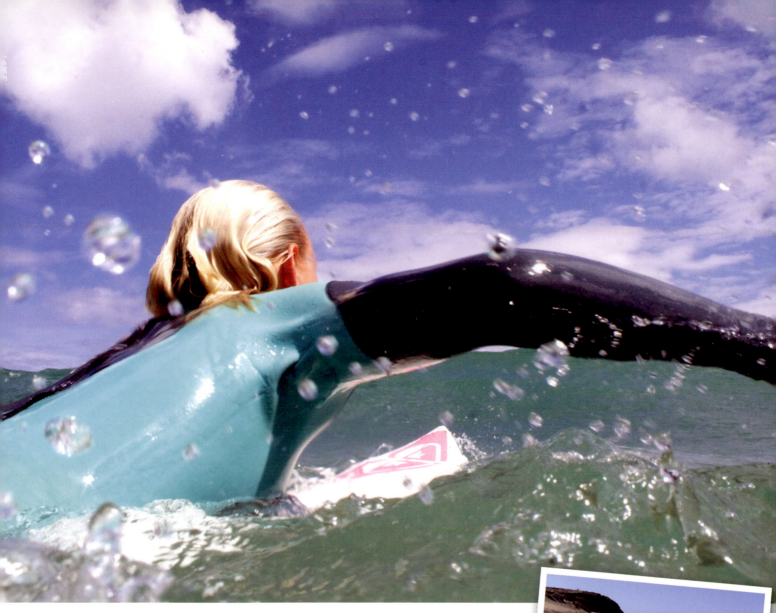

PADDLING OUT

To paddle your board, lie on it so the board's nose is just clear of the surface of the water. Paddle using a swimming 'crawl' stroke and keep your head up to see where you're going. After 10 minutes of this you'll probably be in agony! The reason for this is that you don't yet have strong enough back and shoulder muscles to maintain the paddling action. But don't worry, you'll develop them pretty quickly if you're in the water often enough. If you don't get in all that often, then a few lengths of the local pool will definitely help.

Paddling out through line-after-line of whitewater is hard work. With practise, you'll find that the key to paddling is to use a steady rhythm. Don't paddle flat out; go at a steady pace and save some energy for the occasional burst of speed you'll need to get over – or under – a big set. To catch your first waves it's essential to paddle, then you wait for a wave with the nose pointing towards the shore and dive onto the board in a similar way that you would leap onto a sledge to go down a snowy hill.

Advanced surfers use a technique called duck-diving to get under the waves, but beginners' boards are generally too buoyant for this. Instead you need to paddle hard towards the wave, shift your weight back so the nose of the board lifts up just before the wave reaches you, then let the wave pass underneath you.

GETTING TO YOUR FEET: BEST FOOT FORWARD!

THERE ARE THREE POPULAR TECHNIQUES TO GET TO YOUR FEET. CHOOSE THE ONE THAT SUITS YOU BEST:

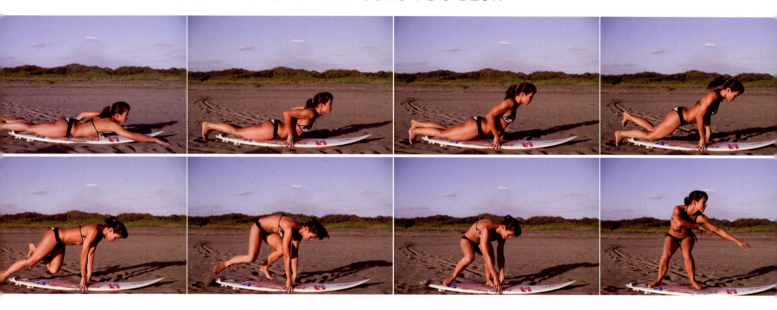

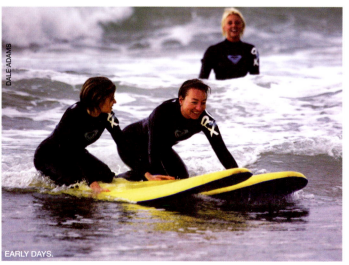

DALE ADAMS

EARLY DAYS.

TECHNIQUE 1: JUMP TO IT!

Position your hands under your chest flat on the deck of the board with your arms out the side like chicken wings - the more bent they are the more upward push you'll get. Push yourself into a standing position in one smooth movement. It's the same movement as a squat thrust but with a turn in it, so that your hips come up side ways. Make sure that you push off both hands equally so that you don't un balance one side of the board before the other. Lead with your front foot and aim to keep central in order to keep the board stable. You should try to get your weight on your front foot as quickly as possible.

Assume the surfing stance!

Your feet should be slightly wider than your shoulder distance apart, assume a crouched position, with a low centre of gravity for balance. Keep your back straight and try to keep your nose in line with your knee and your big toe. Stand with your back foot at 90 degrees to the board's stringer (central line), and your front foot at about 45 degrees. Don't stand like a ballet dancer, you need to be side on with your shoulders running length ways up the board. Look where you're going, not at your feet! Your arms should be held up at about shoulder height to help your balance like a tightrope walker. It's essential to look in the direction that you're aiming to go, this will keep your head up and stop you putting too much weight too far forward.

TECHNIQUE 2: STEP TO IT

If you find it too difficult to get to your feet in one movement you can do it in two or three steps. Ultimately it is much better to get up in one movement but this is a good way to get you stood up until you can manage it.

After you have definitely caught the wave you need to bring both of your knees forward until you're in a kneeling position with your hands holding on to the rails of the board. When you feel that you have good enough balance bring your front foot round the side of the rail and plant it in front of you in the middle of the board. You'll need to allow your leg to come through by moving the relevant hand off the rail.

Now hold the rails again with your hands to maintain your balance. Now as smoothly as possible, turn your hips and stand up, putting your weight on your front foot. It's really important to look towards the beach, don't look down. As soon as both feet are flat on the board assume the surfing stance as described in Technique 1.

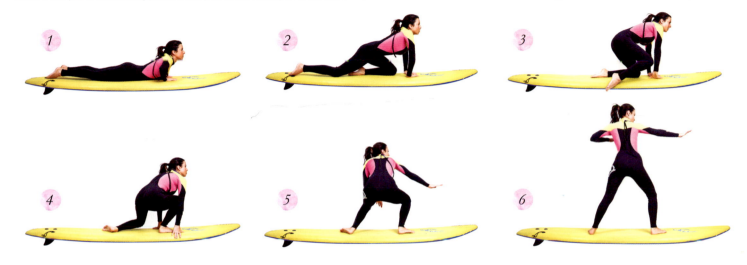

TECHNIQUE 3: ONE KNEE, ONE FOOT

If you find it easier, the one foot, one knee method will see you bring your back leg up on to the board first, placing your knee in the centre of the stringer line. Then when you have your balance, bring your other leg around the side of the rail and plant it in front of you. Keep your hands on the rail and steady yourself. When you are comfortable, look up, twist your hips and place your back foot on the board. Stand slowly until you are in a crouch and keep your arms up to keep you balance.

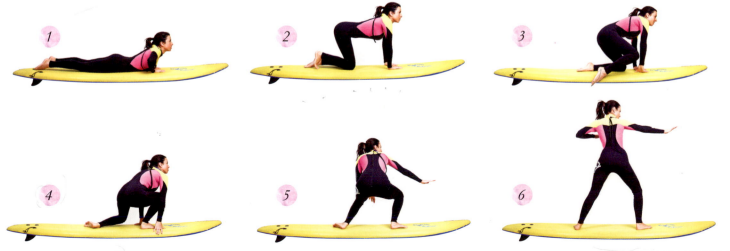

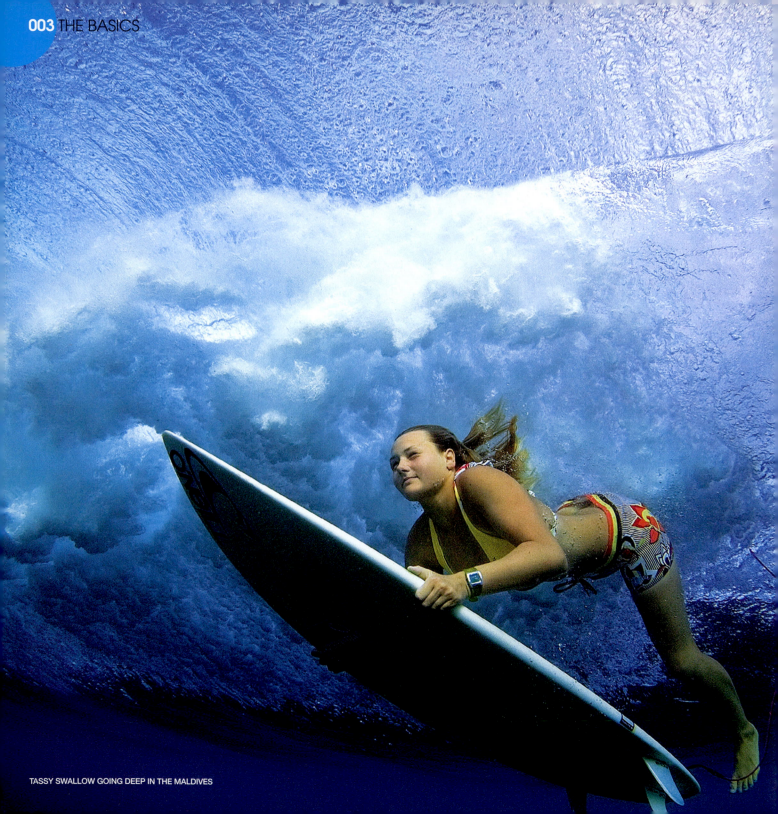

TASSY SWALLOW GOING DEEP IN THE MALDIVES

CATCHING WHITEWATER WAVES

Select a whitewater (broken) wave about 10 yards away from where you are. Swing your board around so it's pointing at the beach, jump on, and get into the paddling position. Make sure no-one else is already riding the wave, and that there's no-one in your way. When the wave is five yards away, start paddling as hard as you can. You'll need to do at least six strokes to catch it. Keep glancing behind, so you know when the wave is about to reach you. Next, if you've timed it correctly, you'll feel yourself lifted up and pushed forward by the wave. Now comes the hard part: getting to your feet.

Once you've finished your ride don't just run up onto the sand as this might damage your fins. Just step off the side of the board and you'll stop. Never dive off your board!

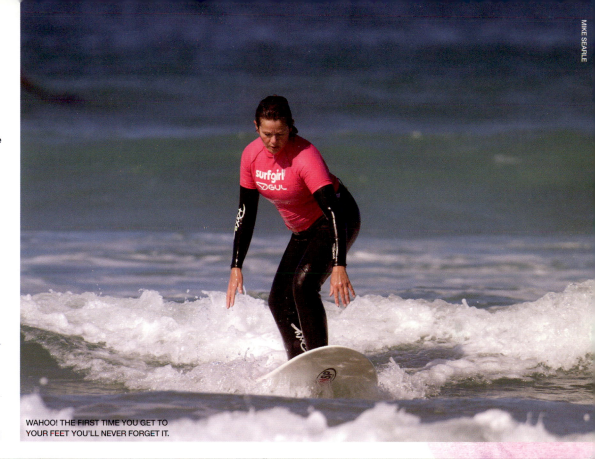

WAHOO! THE FIRST TIME YOU GET TO YOUR FEET YOU'LL NEVER FORGET IT.

MIKE SEARLE

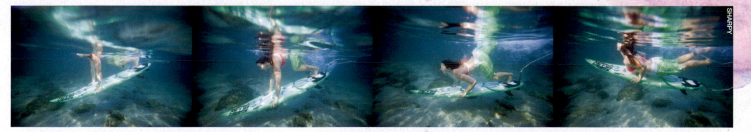

SHARPY

DUCKDIVING

Duckdiving can be almost as hard to master as standing up, and requires a lot of practice to get right. In reality you need to be on a smaller board to truly get under waves, but even on a larger board you can prevent yourself from getting knocked back too far by duckdiving. Here are 5 steps to the perfect duckdive:

• Paddle with speed towards the whitewater. A duckdive doesn't completely avoid the turbulence from the whitewater, so approaching it with strong forward momentum will minimise how far you get dragged back.

• When you're about two-metres from the wave, place your hands on the rails of your board, just underneath your shoulders. Raise your bum and front leg into the air.

This directs most of your body weight through your arms and therefore sinks the front of your board.

• As you feel the whitewater starting to wash over the top of you, use either your back knee or your back foot to push the tail of your surfboard down. This should completely sink your board and begin to propel it forward under the whitewater.

• Keep driving with your back knee/foot as the whitewater continues to pass over the top of you. You should feel yourself coming back to the surface on the other side of the broken wave.

• You did it! Now keep paddling and repeating until you're through all of the whitewater and out back...

Finally, the key to getting out back quickly is timing. Try to paddle out when you see that a set has almost finished breaking, then go for it.

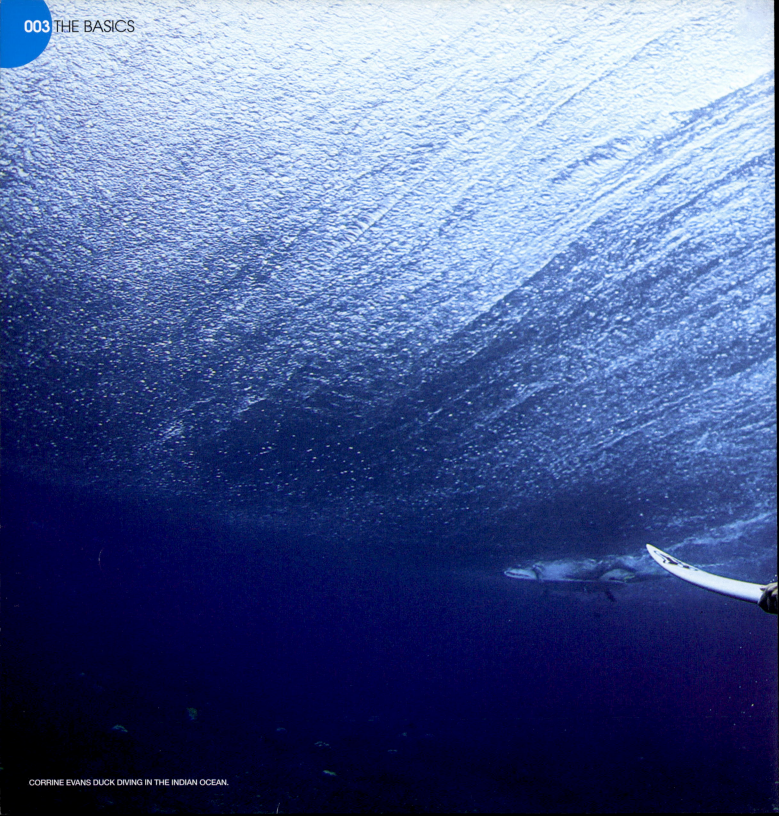

CORRINE EVANS DUCK DIVING IN THE INDIAN OCEAN.

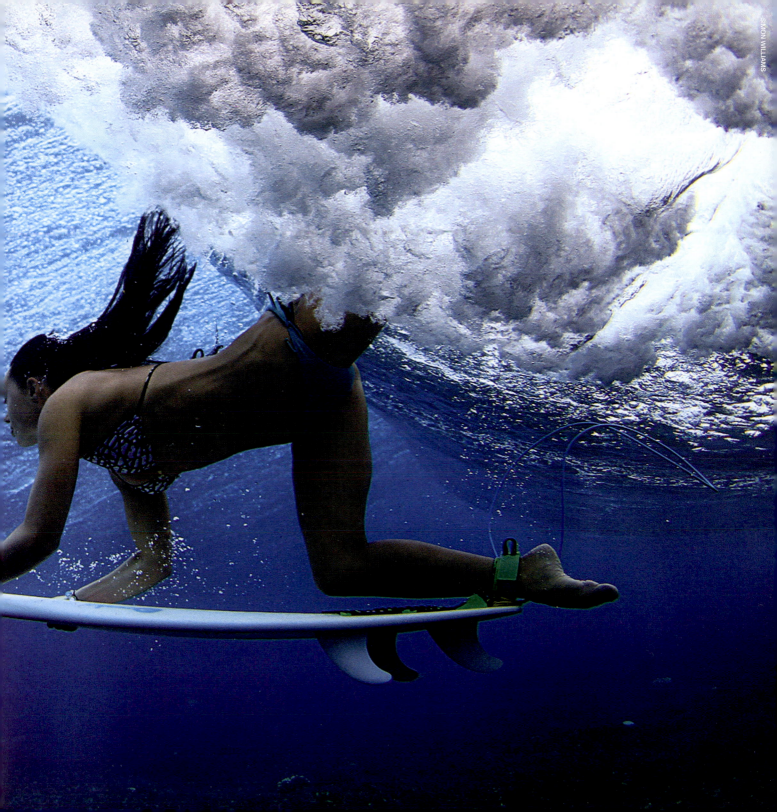

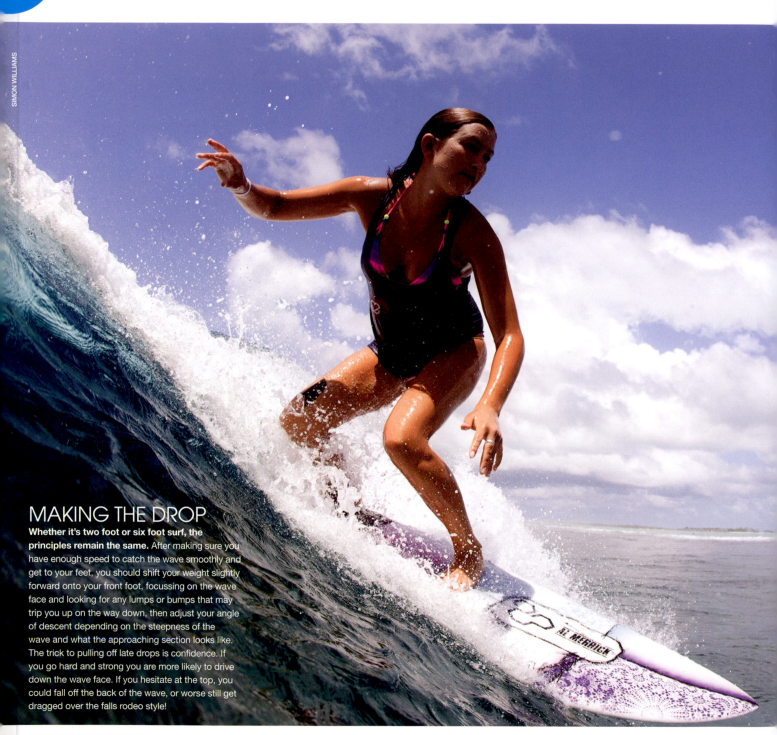

MAKING THE DROP

Whether it's two foot or six foot surf, the principles remain the same. After making sure you have enough speed to catch the wave smoothly and get to your feet, you should shift your weight slightly forward onto your front foot, focussing on the wave face and looking for any lumps or bumps that may trip you up on the way down, then adjust your angle of descent depending on the steepness of the wave and what the approaching section looks like. The trick to pulling off late drops is confidence. If you go hard and strong you are more likely to drive down the wave face. If you hesitate at the top, you could fall off the back of the wave, or worse still get dragged over the falls rodeo style!

CATCHING GREEN WAVES

So now you're out in the lineup and ready to catch some green (unbroken) waves. Before going for one, spend a few minutes watching where the other surfers are taking off and how the waves are breaking. Don't paddle for closeouts – only go for waves which are peeling. Remember to look both ways along a wave before paddling for it – another surfer may already be up and riding.

The technique for catching green waves is similar as the technique for whitewater, except that you need to get to your feet quicker and keep your balance as you drop down the face of the wave. This can make your 'pop' easier (as your board drops away from you it's easier to get your feet on it), but be careful not to lean too far forward as you may nosedive.

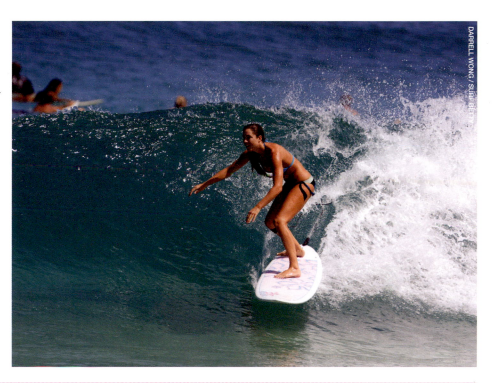

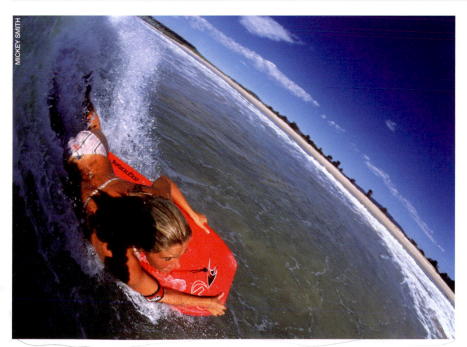

BODYBOARDING

In order to get used to the waves and catch plenty of them, many girls choose to give bodyboarding a try. Just grab a suitably sized board (one that reaches your belly button when it's stood in front of you), get a pair of swim fins and go for it. Any kind of waves can be ridden, and the board is soft so you don't have to worry about being hit by it. Plus it's smaller and lighter so it's easier to lug around, and it's easier to paddle out. Within a few sessions you should be proficient enough to paddle outback into the line up, catch unbroken waves and 'trim' along.

Bodyboarding provides easily achievable goals, plus it's easier to keep your balance, and you get a great sensation of speed as you're closer to the wave. Check out the ThreeSixty Bodyboard Manual for more information about the sport, available from www.orcashop.co.uk

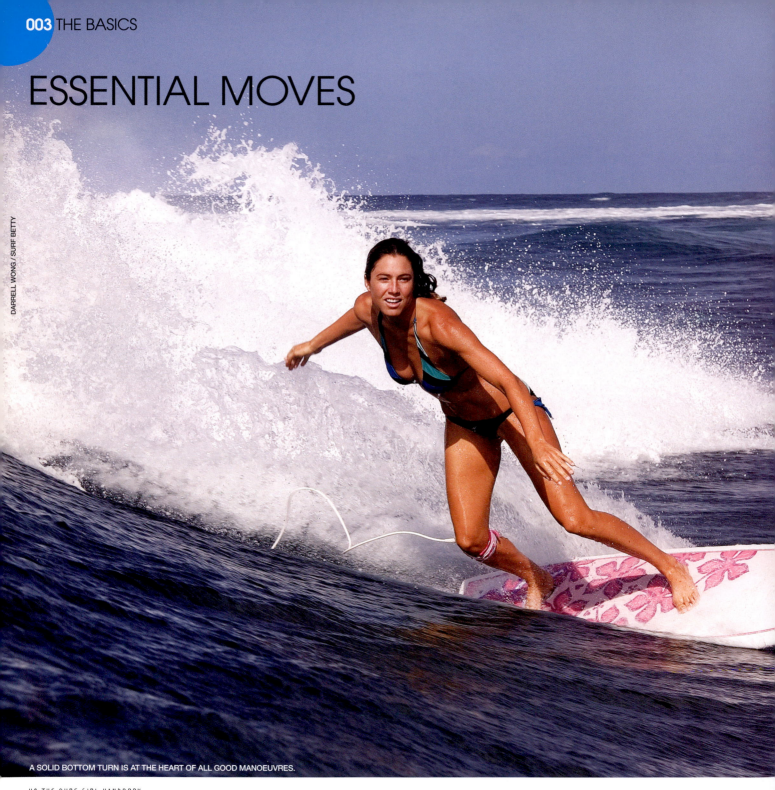

ESSENTIAL MOVES

DARRELL WONG / SURF BETTY

A SOLID BOTTOM TURN IS AT THE HEART OF ALL GOOD MANOEUVRES.

BOTTOM TURN

The bottom turn is the first and most important manoeuvre every surfer should learn. As you drop into the wave, the idea is to transfer your weight smoothly to the inside rail and turn the board along the wave. To do this, put more weight through your back foot and turn your board towards the wave face, keeping your knees bent, until your board is facing along the wave face. A good bottom turn converts the momentum gained from the take-off into the speed necessary to continue down the line, or into the next manoeuvre.

Advanced surfers will often carve smooth, low centre-of-gravity turns in order to generate maximum speed.

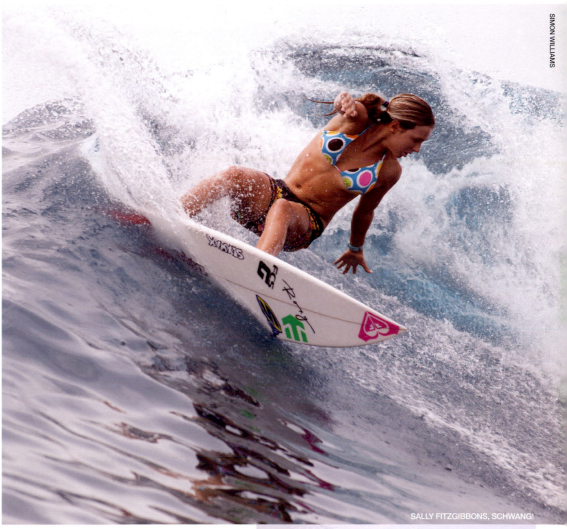

SALLY FITZGIBBONS, SCHWANG!

CUTBACK

This basic manoeuvre enables you to change direction and return to the steepest part of the breaking wave, the pocket, without any loss of speed. There are several varieties of cutbacks, from simple carves through to full figure-of-eight manoeuvres ('roundhouse cutbacks') – the type you can perform will depend on the wave's shape and power. Small mushy waves require small snappy cutbacks to retain maximum speed. Large powerful waves allow the surfer to go way out onto the shoulder of the wave, then accelerate through a large powerful turn back into the pocket, before slashing back around onto the wave face.

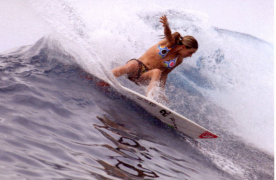

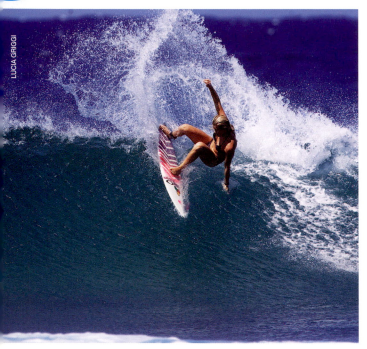

LUCIA GRIGGI

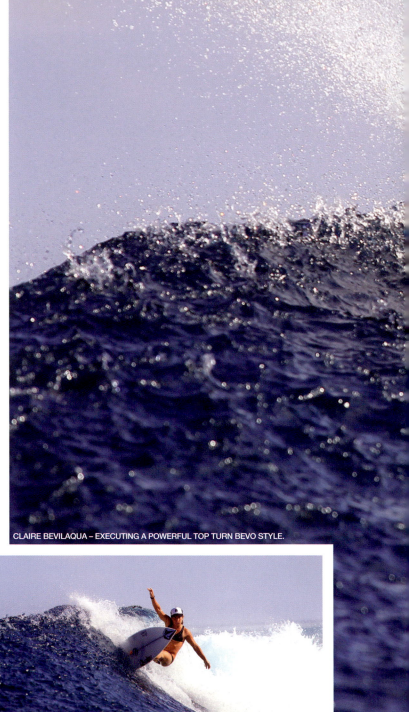

BOTTOM TURN INTO TOP TURN

The vertical top turn is a more critical version of the basic top turn, performed on the steepest section of the wave. To set up the manoeuvre you need to do a good wide bottom turn, then project your board vertically up the wave face, aiming at the steepest part of the unbroken lip. As you reach the apex of the turn, twist your head and shoulders towards the bottom of the wave, and your board will follow, snapping tightly off the top. (Look towards the pocket of the wave, not at your board.) As you drop down the wave again, you'll pick up momentum for the next manoeuvre.

CLAIRE BEVILAQUA – EXECUTING A POWERFUL TOP TURN BEVO STYLE.

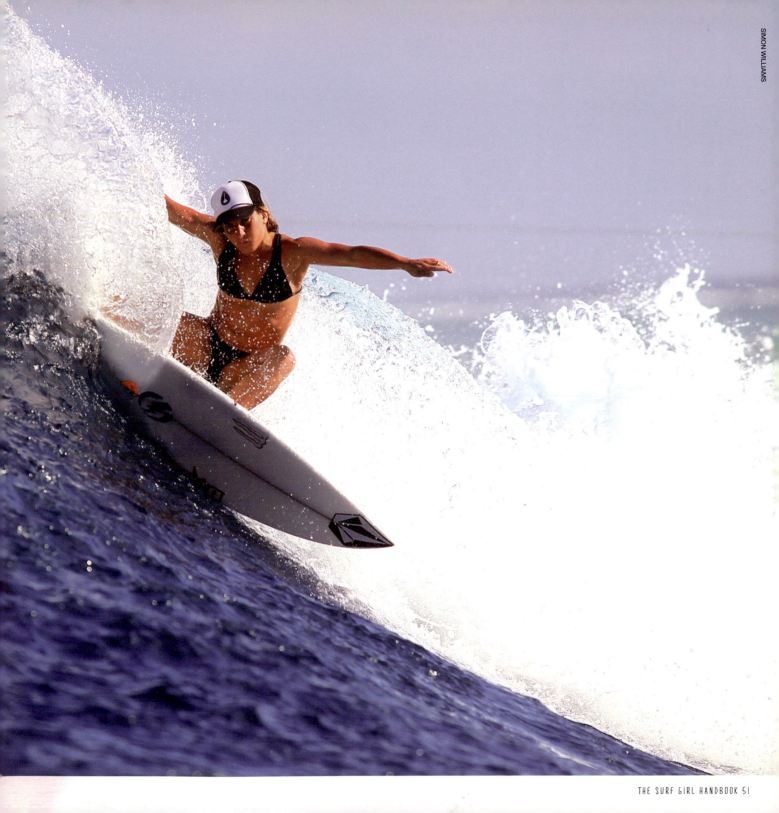

WIPING OUT

Wiping out is an intrinsic part of surfing, and you'd might as well roll with the punches. It's the ocean's karma – you get some good ones, and you get a flogging. But how do you deal with a wipeout?

The fear of wiping out is natural, but you have to learn to deal with it. Most wipeouts last just five or ten seconds, unless you're into some big, powerful waves! Most people can hold their breath easily in a pool for about 30 seconds. The problem is that you don't think you can last out when you're being thrown around by a wave. You're underwater, you can't see or hear anything and all that water around you is disorientating and scary. There's one thing you really need to do, and it ain't easy: let go and realise you just can't fight it. If you just relax then you will come up.

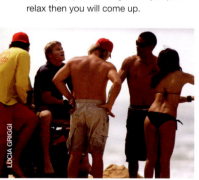

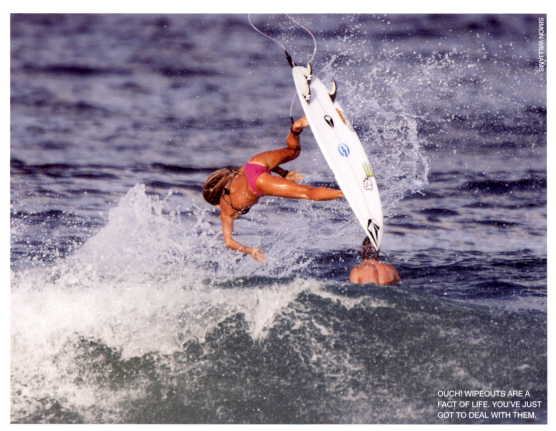

OUCH! WIPEOUTS ARE A FACT OF LIFE. YOU'VE JUST GOT TO DEAL WITH THEM.

SIMON WILLIAMS

LUCIA GRIGGI

HERE'S SOME TIPS TO REMEMBER NEXT TIME YOU TAKE A HIT.

1. You might have some forewarning that you're coming off and if so try to jump away from your board or push it away with your feet. (But never do this if your board might injure someone else in the water and never dive off headfirst in shallow water.)

2. Protect your head. If you think it's in danger (from the bottom, your board, or the goatboater who dropped in on you!) then tuck yourself up into a ball to avoid getting hurt and when you resurface, protect your head from stray boards.

3. If you just have a split second 'oh, crickey…' moment before you're hurled into the pit then all you can do is take a deep breath and try to notice what's happening around you. Having some idea of how many waves are behind you in the set, how far away the next one is, where other people are and where your board is will help once you come up. While you're down though: just relax and suck it up!

4. Don't panic. You'll use up your oxygen faster, and it won't get you anywhere. You will be frightened plenty of times when you surf, but you have to recognise that you can't be in total control of the situation.

5. There are things you can do to help you deal with wipeouts. Firstly, get out there. Swim, surf, bodysurf, bodyboard and experience the power of waves and learn about how they break. Get used to the power of the ocean. Watch other people and how they fall off different boards and different waves. Fitness is also important – when you're tired, you struggle more to catch your breath and get back on the board. So you need to improve your cardiovascular fitness – swimming is one of the best things to do, as is paddling practice. Yoga helps with controlling your breathing and staying calm and focused.

6. Getting off a wave: If you're on a whitewater wave, there's not much power left in it as it's already broken, so just pop off away from your board and wait until you come up. If you're on a green wave try to dive through the back or as deep as you can to avoid the worst of the breaking wave's power. If it's small enough you might be able to jump over the back.

ROCK ENTRY

GETTING THERE...

Entry to some breaks (particularly point or reef breaks) may require a sketchy clamber across slimy dangerous rocks. It's easy to fall over, so the key is to concentrate on where every foot is going to be placed, and to use your spare hand for balance. Think about where your next foot is going, and plan a few steps ahead. As with surfing, keeping your centre of gravity low by crouching down can also go a long way to helping you stay upright.

GETTING IN

Once you've successfully negotiated the walk across the rocks, the next stage – entering the water – can be equally tricky.

1. The key is to locate a ledge of rock with a drop-off into the deepest possible area of water. Watch the spot for a couple of sets and when the water recedes (just after a wave has washed in and it washes out again) check the area for dangerous looking exposed rocks.

2. When you find a safe entry point, wait for a wave to come towards you – the last wave of a set is best. Time your leap so that you jump over the foam and land on the back of the wave as it's coming towards you. It is essential to keep the board pointing out towards the horizon so that it creates the least resistance to the oncoming wave as possible. If you hesitate, then wait for the next wave and try again. Do not jump into the water as the wave begins to drain back out to sea again, as the water will be at its most shallow at this point and you'll literally hit rock bottom.

3. Your leap needs to be well-timed, committed and your board needs to be under your body. That way, if the worst happens, at least you will land on your board on top of a rock instead of impaling yourself!

6. As you hit the water, start paddling for the horizon. If it's shallow then don't put your arms in too deep – just stroke out with your arms – and if you've waited for the last wave of a set then there should be a relatively easy paddle and you're away, and no duck diving: hooray!

Note: Never enter the water without knowing where you plan to exit it from. It can be a lot harder to get out than to get in!

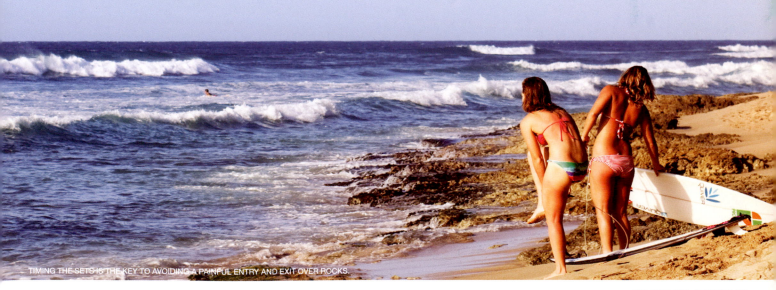

TIMING THE SETS IS THE KEY TO AVOIDING A PAINFUL ENTRY AND EXIT OVER ROCKS.

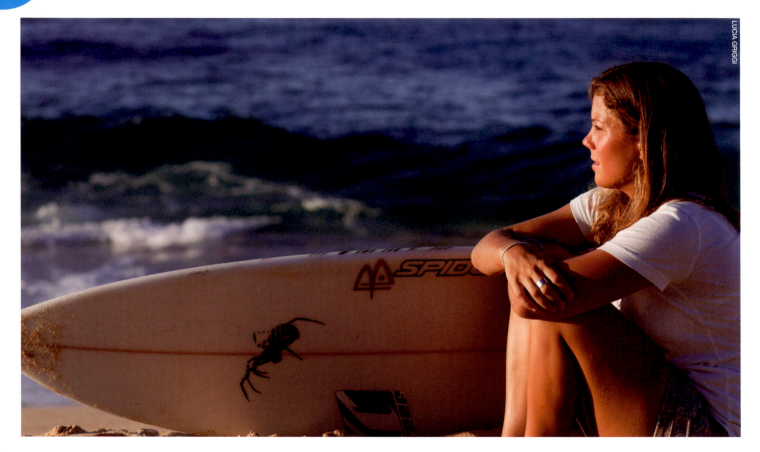

LUCIA GRIGGI

BEING WAVE SAVVY
THE SECRET TO CATCHING MORE WAVES IS IN TIMING AND WAVE KNOWLEDGE.

1. First up check the tide before you head off. This is important as the waves that are closing out now may fire on a low tide bank in an hour or two, or that fat, slow wave might turn into a fun shorey come high tide. You need to know what the best conditions for the break are. The best source of this information is local surfers – they know all about the potential hazards at the beach too, as well as what turns it on and off.

2. Time the sets. Otherwise you'll spend your whole session battling against them and wear yourself out. If you know how often sets are coming in then you can time your paddle so you get out in between them. Watch at least two sets going through before you get in, so that you can gauge the size of the surf and where

the sets are working best.

3. Before you start paddling out, watch other surfers. If they're getting out back quickly then follow them. If they're getting nailed maybe you need to move to another part of the beach. Also, try to avoid crowds, even if it means walking further down the beach – it'll be worth it as you'll end up getting more waves.

4. Once you're out back make sure you're in the right place. To start with, line up two markers on the beach so you can gauge your position and avoid being dragged off the peak. Next, make sure you're in the right zone – not too far in and not too far out. This is one

of the most difficult things that surfers have to learn and it only comes with experience. The best tip is to watch where everyone else is taking off and follow suit. Longboarders stay further out the back than shortboarders so position yourself accordingly. Once a set has come through you should have your position sussed.

5. Once you're ready to catch a wave, only go for waves that will peel. If a wave's getting steep all across its length at the same time it's likely to close out. Once you're in position, make sure that you have enough paddling speed to catch the wave, angle your board a little so that you don't head straight down and you're away!

Stay motivated

We don't all live in tropical climes, unfortunately, and for those of us less fortunate winter can be a harsh time. The water's cold, daylight's limited, the amount of kit that you need is ridiculous, and getting changed in freezing temperatures is a shivering nightmare.

Surfing at the weekends is often the only option, so keeping your focus and motivation can be difficult – especially if for a couple of weekends in a row the waves are slack or the wind's wrong and you don't end up getting in.

So, how do you keep surfing all year and maintain your performance? Check out the following techniques to help you stay on top of your game and fend off those winter blues.

GO FOR GOALS

Goal-setting is a great way to maintain drive in any sport. Surfing differs slightly from the likes of football and athletics because most of us don't partake in it to be competitive or win anything, but goal setting will help you to improve your surfing. Set yourself motivational goals like aiming to surf at least four times a week, or practical ones like learning roundhouse cutback in the next four months! Having a target to achieve will increase your motivation and give you heaps of satisfaction when you achieve your goal.

GET PSYCHED!

Watch DVDs before you leave the house and focus on the moves that surfers are busting. There's no reason why you can't pull moves like that! Sure you've got more rubber on, but that's no excuse...

Getting amped to music also helps to focus you and psyche you up for your next session. Some people use thrashy punk stuff whilst others find that more laid-back Moby-style stuff works for them. Music can be that crucial bit of leverage to get you out of the car on those frosty earlies. There is no excuse for planning to go surfing, getting a crew together and then bottling it at the last minute because of the cold. You'll just regret it later, and it may be the last chance you get to surf for the next few weeks.

SHORT SHARP BURSTS

In summer it's easy to surf for hours, but in the winter you get colder quicker which – aside from being generally unpleasant – will affect your ability to perform. Go for shorter sessions and aim to catch more waves and bust more moves. Time your session to get the best out of the tide, wind and crowd conditions. If you make sure that you've got a dry wetsuit to jump into it'll be much easier to get moving and, after your session, try to hang your wetsuit somewhere warm and dry, or – worst case – leave it in a black bin-bag in the winter sun!

As soon as you get out of the car and are greeted with the cold, go for a gentle jog and stretch to warm yourself up. Then pull your suit on as quickly as you can and get out there. Study the break and use channels and rips to plan the paddle out route needing the least amount of duckdives. If you're using a beach not too far from home then get some decent seat covers so that you can drive home in your wettie and get changed in the warm.

CORRECT KIT

If you've got wetsuit boots with holes in them, or a wettie that lets water leak down the back, you'll dread hitting the water even more. Christmas marks the beginning of the coldest stretch of winter in the northern hemisphere, so a good time to ask for gloves, hoods and boots from Santa!

Having the best kit is going to help you combat (and enjoy!) the worst elements that Mother Nature can throw at you. Check out the season's best wetties, and get the one that fits you the best. Go on: treat yourself!

MIKE SEARLE

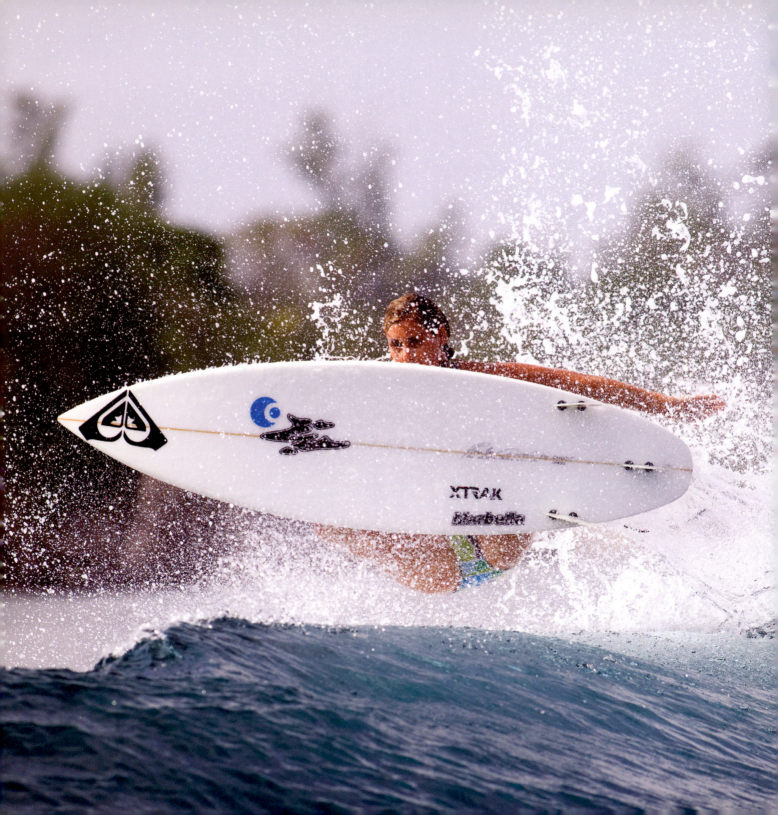

LUCIA GRICCI

TURN UP THE HEAT

chapter four

NOW YOU'VE GOT THE BASICS DOWN, IT'S TIME TO STEP THINGS UP, SO LET'S
TAKE A LOOK AT SOME OF THE MANOEUVRES GUARANTEED TO TURN HEADS AT YOUR
LOCAL BEACH. AND ONCE YOU START TO PUSH YOURSELF HARDER PHYSICALLY,
YOU'LL FIND THAT YOU NEED A MORE FOCUSSED MINDSET, SO WE ALSO LOOK AT
SOME CONFIDENCE BOOSTING TIPS FOR TACKLING BIGGER WAVES.

FLOATERS AND AIRS

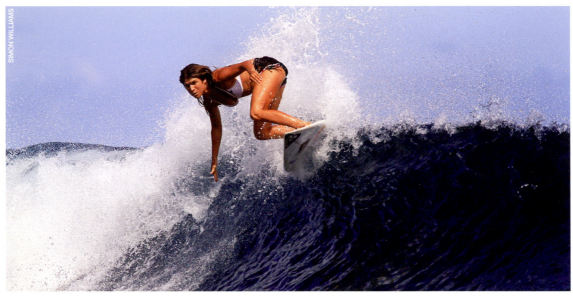

SIMON WILLIAMS

FLOATERS

The floater re-entry was one of the hottest moves of the 80s and is now a standard manoeuvre for most advanced surfers.
The basic floater is performed by steering your board up onto the breaking lip with enough speed to glide along it for some distance, before dropping down the curtain of the wave and continuing the ride. Floaters, like aerials, are 'horizontal' manoeuvres: you set them up by pumping down the line, doing a shallow bottom-turn, and gliding up onto the lip at maximum speed. Then it's just a matter of committing yourself and steering out of the lip, so that you freefall back down into the trough of the wave.

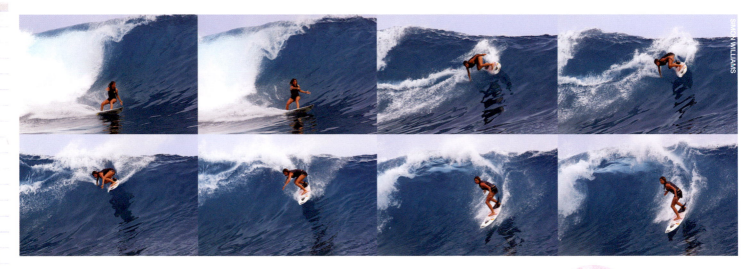

SIMON WILLIAMS

BACKHAND OFF THE TOP

The key to a good strong backhand off the lip begins with the bottom turn. Open your body shape by pulling your inside shoulder towards the wave and look to the point you want to hit. As your shoulders turn whip the board through with your legs and move your weight on to your back foot. About three quarters of the way up the wave face you should feel ready to head back down. Turn your head and shoulders back down the wave face and whip the board back under your body. The amount of spray you throw is directly related to the power you put into the snap!

Top tip
Take aim! Look where you want to go. It sounds weird but if you're head is pointing in the direction, the shoulders and then the rest of the body will follow.

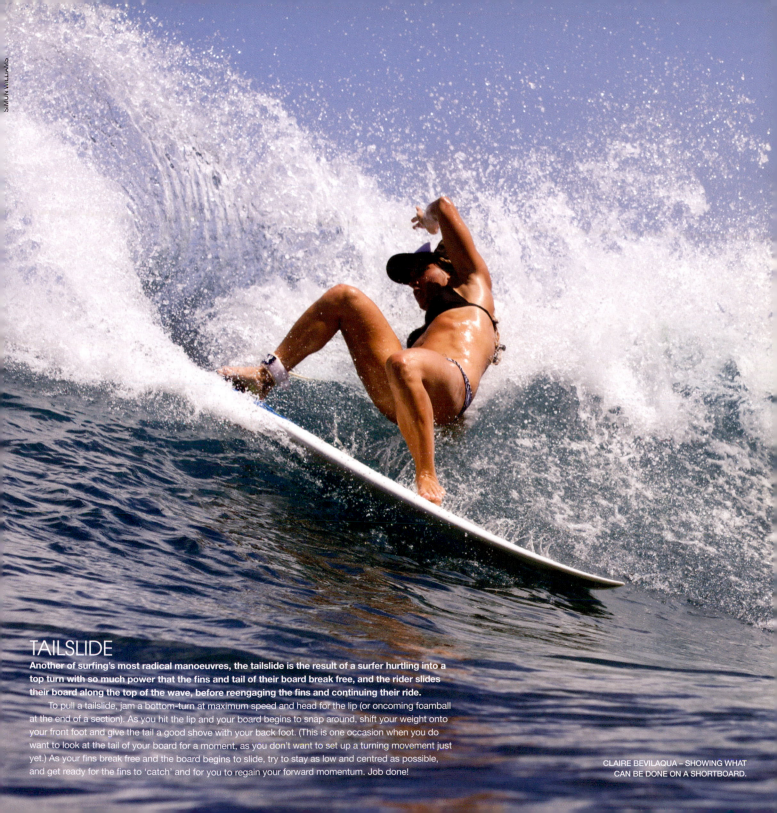

TAILSLIDE

Another of surfing's most radical manoeuvres, the tailslide is the result of a surfer hurtling into a top turn with so much power that the fins and tail of their board break free, and the rider slides their board along the top of the wave, before reengaging the fins and continuing their ride.

To pull a tailslide, jam a bottom-turn at maximum speed and head for the lip (or oncoming foamball at the end of a section). As you hit the lip and your board begins to snap around, shift your weight onto your front foot and give the tail a good shove with your back foot. (This is one occasion when you do want to look at the tail of your board for a moment, as you don't want to set up a turning movement just yet.) As your fins break free and the board begins to slide, try to stay as low and centred as possible, and get ready for the fins to 'catch' and for you to regain your forward momentum. Job done!

CLAIRE BEVILAQUA – SHOWING WHAT
CAN BE DONE ON A SHORTBOARD.

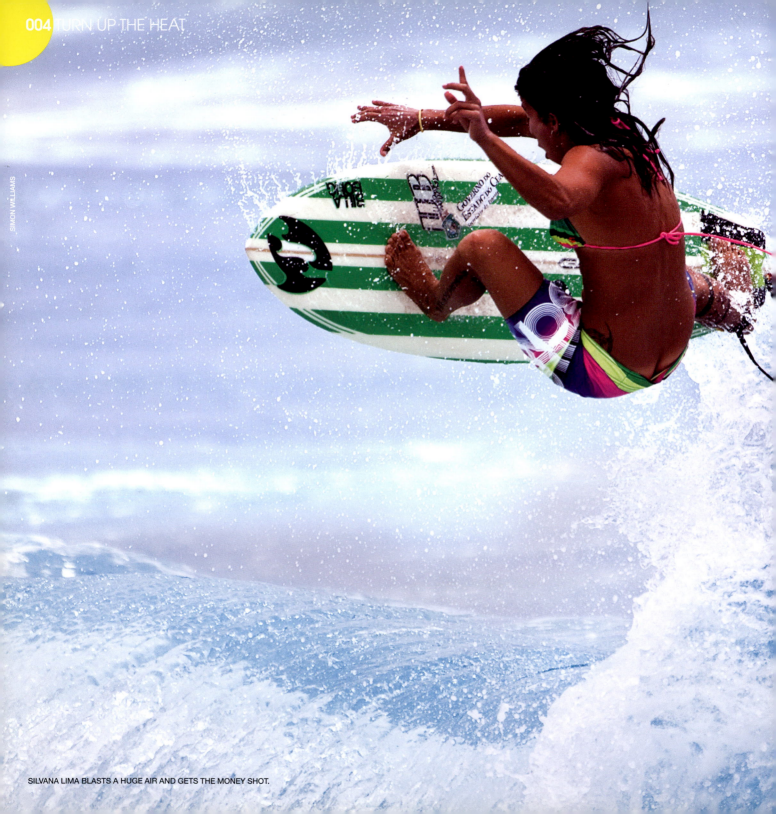

SIMON WILLIAMS

SILVANA LIMA BLASTS A HUGE AIR AND GETS THE MONEY SHOT.

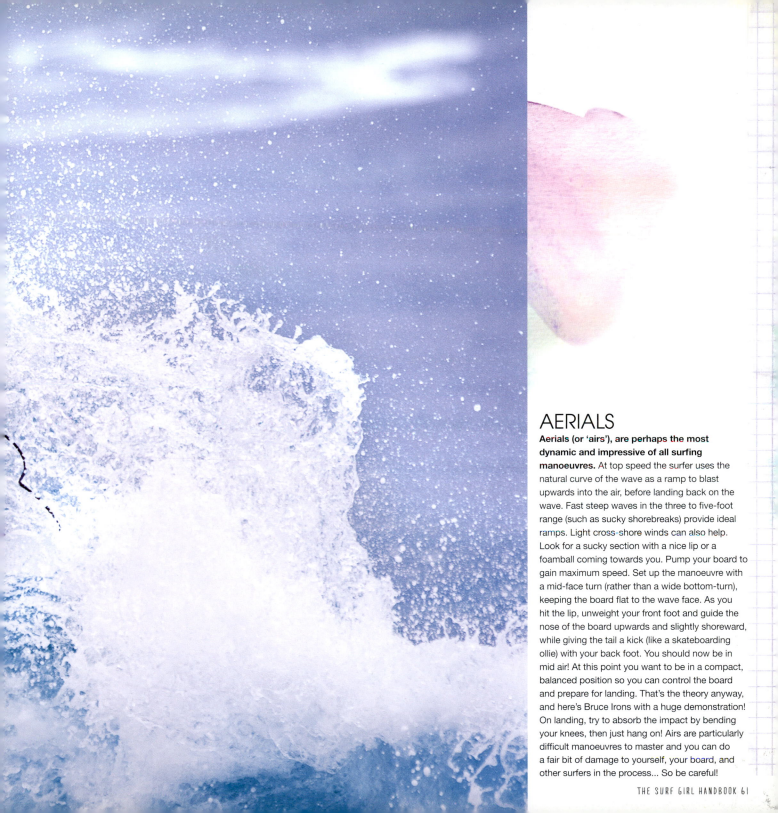

AERIALS

Aerials (or 'airs'), are perhaps the most dynamic and impressive of all surfing manoeuvres. At top speed the surfer uses the natural curve of the wave as a ramp to blast upwards into the air, before landing back on the wave. Fast steep waves in the three to five-foot range (such as sucky shorebreaks) provide ideal ramps. Light cross-shore winds can also help. Look for a sucky section with a nice lip or a foamball coming towards you. Pump your board to gain maximum speed. Set up the manoeuvre with a mid-face turn (rather than a wide bottom-turn), keeping the board flat to the wave face. As you hit the lip, unweight your front foot and guide the nose of the board upwards and slightly shoreward, while giving the tail a kick (like a skateboarding ollie) with your back foot. You should now be in mid air! At this point you want to be in a compact, balanced position so you can control the board and prepare for landing. That's the theory anyway, and here's Bruce Irons with a huge demonstration! On landing, try to absorb the impact by bending your knees, then just hang on! Airs are particularly difficult manoeuvres to master and you can do a fair bit of damage to yourself, your board, and other surfers in the process... So be careful!

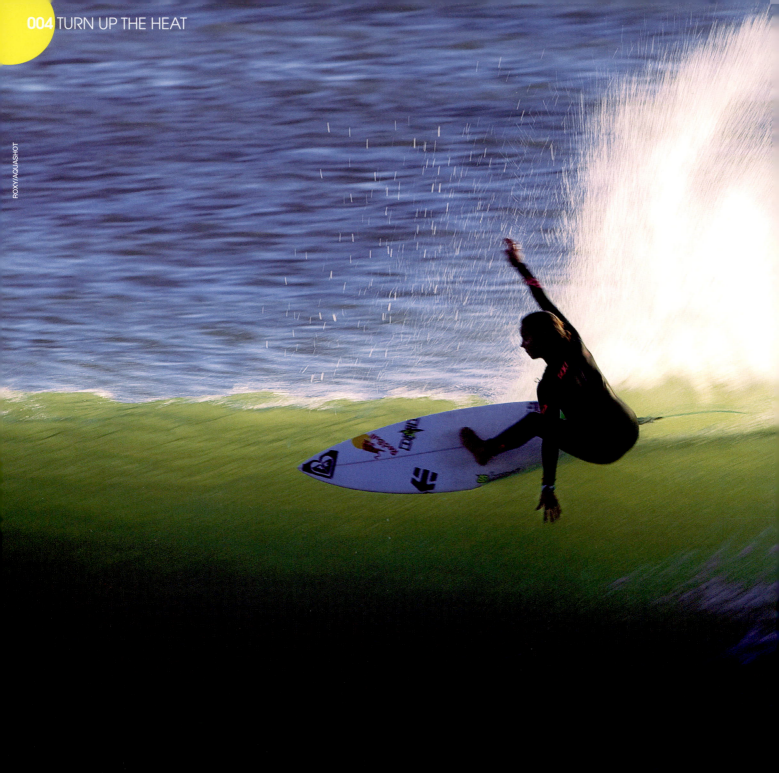

ROXY/AQUASHOT

SALLY FITZGIBBONS SPEEDING DOWN THE LINE

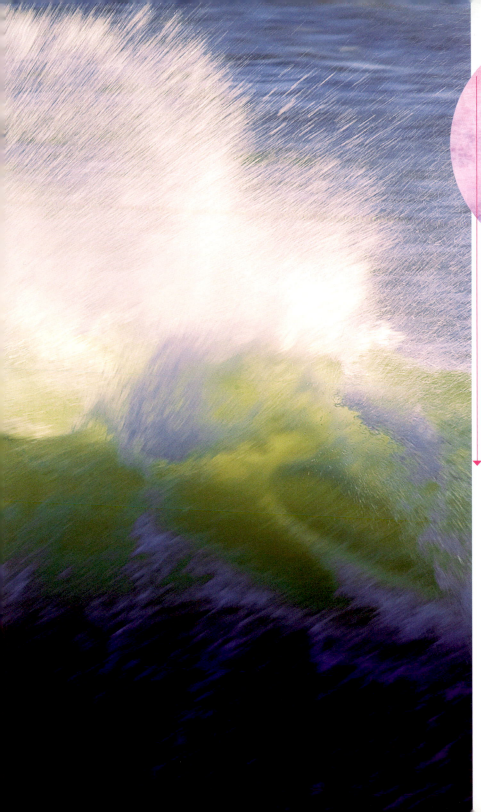

PRO TIPS

with SALLY FITZGIBBONS

GO FASTER!

Speed is a very important factor and is the major ingredient when wanting to do any manoeuvre. To go faster you must energise with your arms – throw both arms up to around shoulder height and in the direction you want to go. Once you have achieved that initial lift off, you want to weave your board on the wave face. Little turns up and down the mid face of the wave will see you generating heaps of speed.

To maintain your speed make sure you don't drop too far to the bottom of the wave, or be too far up the face. So between turns, and when you're building your speed and trying to make faster sections, you want to draw your lines nice and smoothly and keep in that speed line mid face. To slow down you must put all your weight on your back foot to stall your board. Doing a turn in the pocket of the wave will also wash off some speed.

Feel what the wave is doing under your feet, practice speeding up and slowing down, and feel what your board naturally wants to do. It's so important to learn to control your speed as every manoeuvre requires a different amount, so find the balance and practice in all types of conditions.

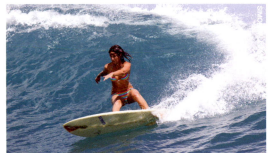

LINKING YOUR MOVES

The more time you spend in the water, the better you learn to read the waves and therefore predict what lies ahead of you and what moves you will be able to link together. Linking moves requires you to think a few steps ahead, so you know as soon as you come out of one turn where you will be heading to next. You must maintain your speed and energy by throwing yourself up and in the direction you want to go. Make sure you fully complete the move you are doing before going into the next to avoid catching a rail.

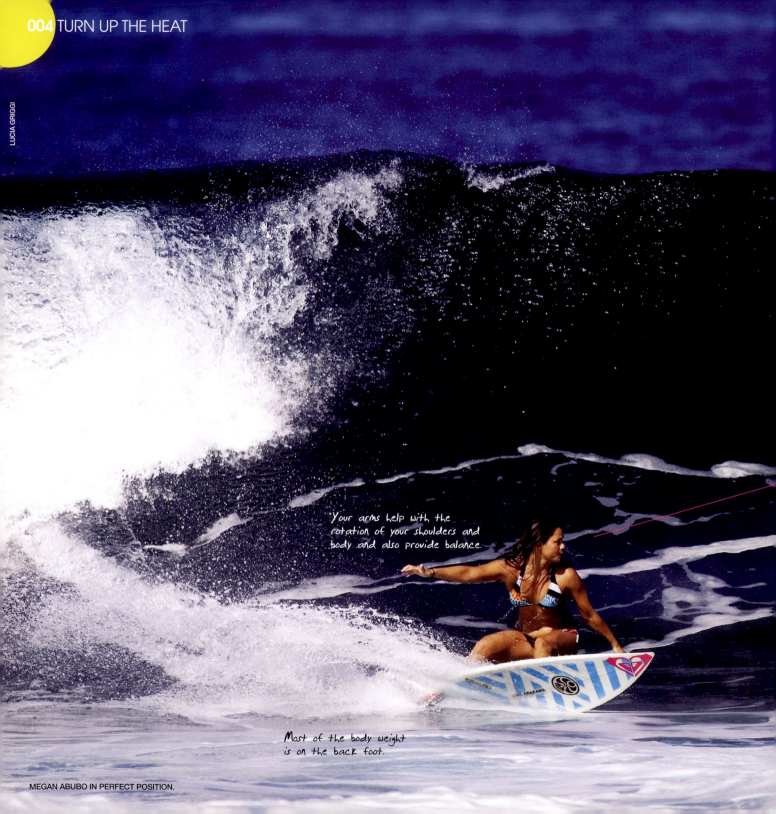

Your arms help with the rotation of your shoulders and body and also provide balance.

Most of the body weight is on the back foot.

MEGAN ABUBO IN PERFECT POSITION.

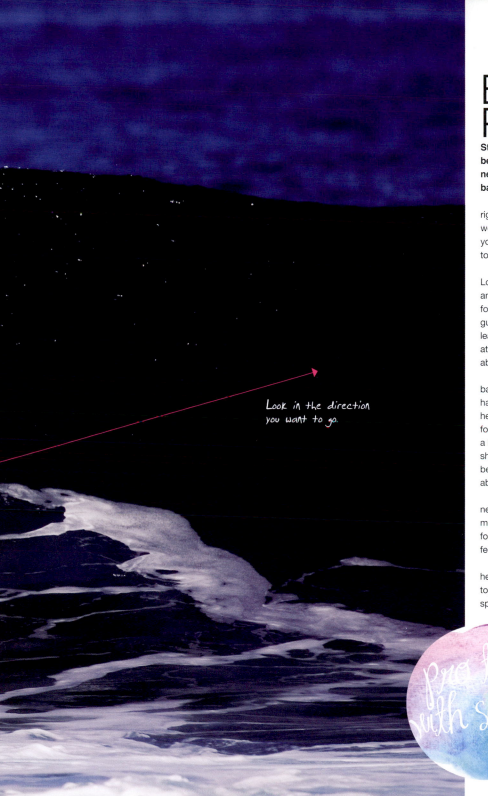

Look in the direction you want to go.

BODY POSITIONING

Stance is the one of the most important ingredients in becoming a good surfer and in ensuring that you can learn new moves. Together with posture, a good stance is the basis for making movements that work.

So, what is a good stance? Firstly, you must get the basics right. Bend at the knees rather than the waist, so that your weight and body stays in a column above your feet. Most of your weight should be on your back foot. To help with this, try to keep the back knee more bent than the front.

Your arms and hands are more important than you think. Loose, floppy arms will lead to floppy surfing. Your arms are an easy connection to your shoulders and the rotation needed for good turns, as well as providing for balance. As a rough guide, your front arm needs to be straight out, slightly bent, but leading over the nose of the board. Your back arm needs to be at about a 90 degree angle, with your hand in front of you just above your waist.

Positioning on the board is crucial. For tight turns, the back foot needs to be right between the fins. Making sure you have a good tail block that you can feel under your back foot helps with this. For down-the-line speed, you need to be more forward on the flatter part of the board. A good tip is to stick a bit of duct tape on the board to mark where your front foot should be. And remember that as you are riding a wave you will be changing what you're doing, so you will need to be thinking about moving your feet, even on a shortboard.

Everybody is built differently and the width of your stance needs to suit your body and board. A wider stance is better for more powerful rail-to-rail surfing, and a narrow stance is great for tight up-and-down surfing, but less so for drive. Find what feels comfortable for you and adjust accordingly.

A good tip is to dig out your surf DVDs and analyse your heroes. There are good and bad stances in there, but all the tops surfers have common characteristics that you'll be able to spot and copy.

pro tips with sally

Making the perfect bottom turn

With your bottom turn you want to drop to the bottom of the wave, then get nice and low to the wave face by leaning on your inside rail, and driving with your legs toward the top of the wave. It should then almost slingshot you upwards. And remember to keep your head looking in the direction you want to go: your board will follow.

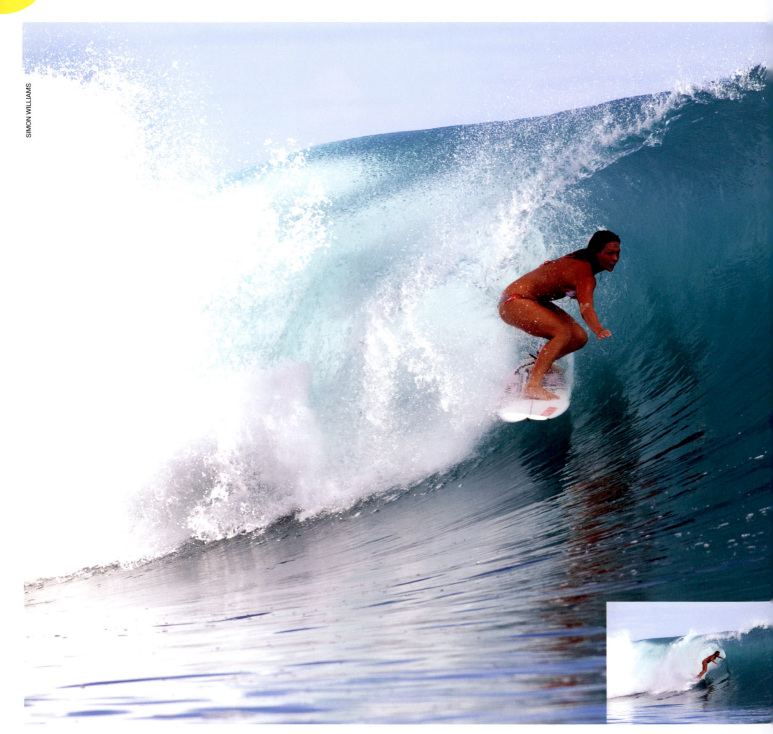

SIMON WILLIAMS

TUBE RIDING

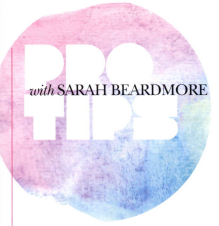

with SARAH BEARDMORE

WQS surfer Sarah Beardmore gives us her pro tips for tube riding.

Tube riding is one of those things that, once you've experienced it, you get a taste for and will have you chasing tubes for ever more! When you come out of your first tube you'll have the confidence to keep practising and hold your position so you get deeper every time.

There are two main ways to tube ride and your options will depend on the wave as well as your positioning. The first is a fast barrel where there is no stalling involved and your weight is kept on your front foot at all times as you race through the section. The second (and probably most common) is where you stall on your back foot to tuck inside the barrel. The sequence shown is an example of this.

Catch a wave and stand up. By this stage, you will recognise if the wave will barrel as it will suck up just behind you or above your head. In this picture I recognised the potential tube and took off on a slight angle to make sure I was able to get in it

as quick as possible.

Look down the line. Slightly bend your knees and turn your body in towards the wave. Drag your arm in the wave if you need to keep your balance. Bend your knees and put weight on your back foot in order to lose speed so you are ready for when the wave curls over your head. Dragging your arm in the wave face can also help.

Crouch down. Just enough so the wave doesn't clip you. Your weight should now be evenly compressed over both legs. Point your front arm out in front of you towards daylight. This helps balance as well as guiding you and your board to where you want to go. Keep crouching low… You're in!

Aim for the light! Start putting weight on your front foot and crouch forward. Your lead arm should still be out. This is where you get ready for your exit and is one of the most crucial parts of barrel riding. The arm is still out and has successfully guided you to where you want to be. It is one thing to feel your first barrel but when you exit that means you have had your first real tube! Keep knees bent and weight on the front foot to gain speed on exit. Hopefully at this stage you have a friend or two whistling at you!

Remain confident and look straight out the tube at all times. If the barrel is fast, you need speed inside it as well as on exit. If you feel the barrel running away from you, remember that it is like any other fast wave – even though you are inside it you still need to gain speed by weaving forward using your legs and throwing your arms forward too. Sometimes it's easy to get over excited, rush the exit and fall off. If you feel like you're losing balance and are going to fall, don't dive toward the crashing part of the wave, try to fall so you go through the back of the wave.

Good luck getting shacked!

SARAH BEARDMORE PULLING INTO THE GREEN ROOM.

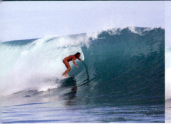
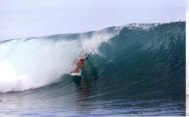
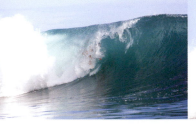
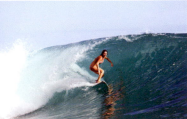

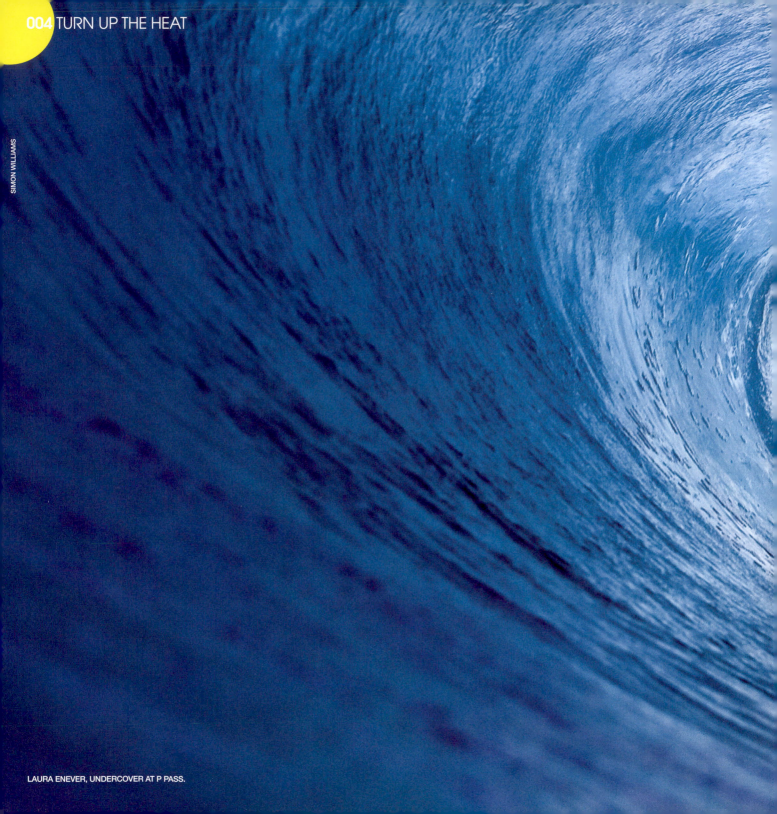

SIMON WILLIAMS

LAURA ENEVER, UNDERCOVER AT P PASS.

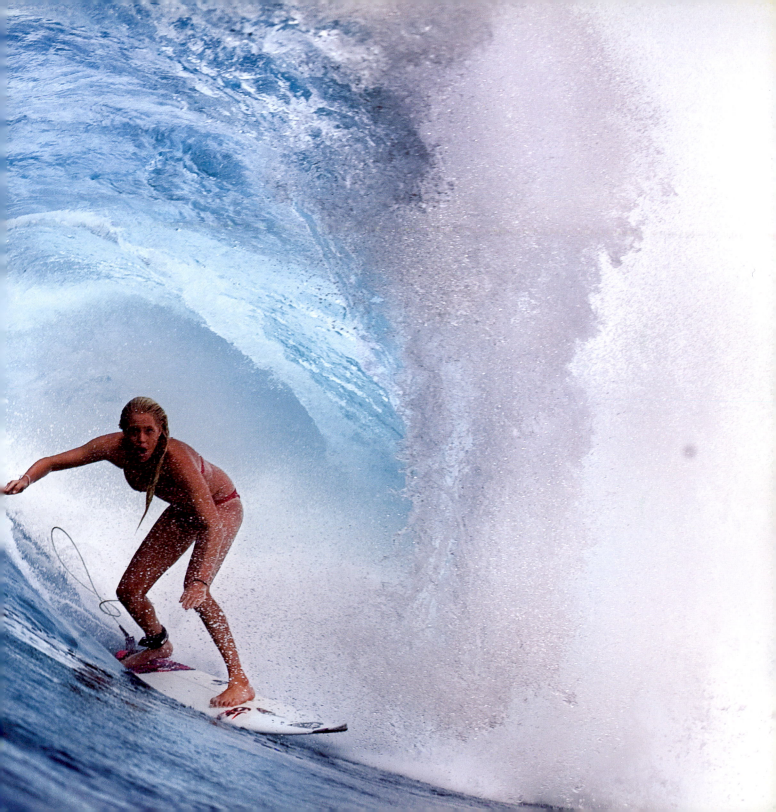

ROXY/HORNBAKER

PUSHING YOUR LIMITS

Becoming a better surfer takes time and is all about challenging yourself — so don't just cruise around chatting away and seeing who's in the lineup next time you're out, surfer Celine Gehret says think about pushing yourself a little bit further.

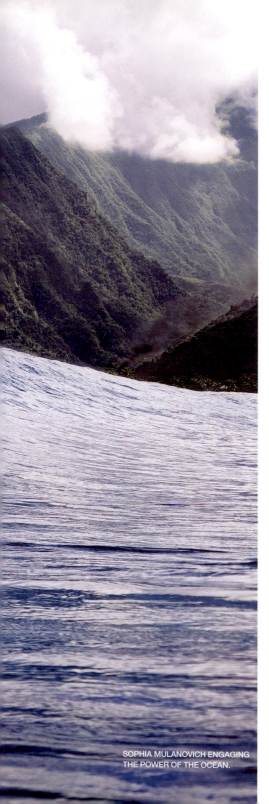

SOPHIA MULANOVICH ENGAGING THE POWER OF THE OCEAN.

1. DON'T BE INTIMIDATED

If you want to push your limits by trying out bigger manoeuvres, then practise them first in surf that you feel really comfortable in – say shoulder-to-head high easy surf at your favourite break. Don't try new and crazy things when you're out of your comfort zone (when the surf's way too big, or you're at a new spot). You don't want to hurt yourself and it will only put you off. Once you're comfortable pulling the move in easy surf, just do the same when it's bigger! And remember that a bigger wave has got more power, so you'll have to put more effort and strength into your turn to pull it off. Don't be intimidated, trust in your ability and go for it!

2. FEEL THE FEAR... AND GO ANYWAY!

How do you know your limits if you don't push them? If you're determined to paddle for that big wave, then do it. Don't hesitate, and never pull back at the last second – that's when the classic 'pulled over' wipeout happens.

Feel and embrace the fear. You'll get a real rush from big drops, and that fear then transforms into pure adrenaline, it's an amazing feeling! When I go for a big wave I think positive, it really works. If you doubt yourself and think that you'll fall, then you probably will. Your ability has a lot to do with your mindset and your attitude, so have a positive attitude and trust in your ability. Once you've made that drop, you'll be buzzing for the next one and it'll feel easier to go for it. And you'll find that big drops are addictive...

3. GET BACK UP AND DO IT AGAIN

If you wipe out then make sure you catch another wave before you leave the water otherwise it can put you off for your next session.

The key to getting your surfing to the next level and going for bigger manoeuvres is to keep going for it. And pushing your limits means falling off a lot – at least to start with. As long as you're prepared and you know where your board is when you fall off then you'll be safe. Remember that it's only water, so (unless you're surfing a super shallow reef break!) you'll be fine!

It's amazing what you can do when you really put your mind to it. The brain is a powerful tool, so use it: Think it, feel it, and next time you're out make sure you push your limits!

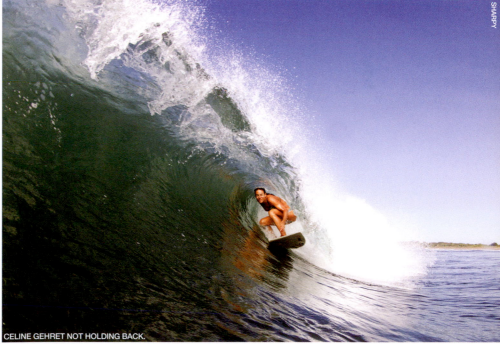

CELINE GEHRET NOT HOLDING BACK.

SHARPY

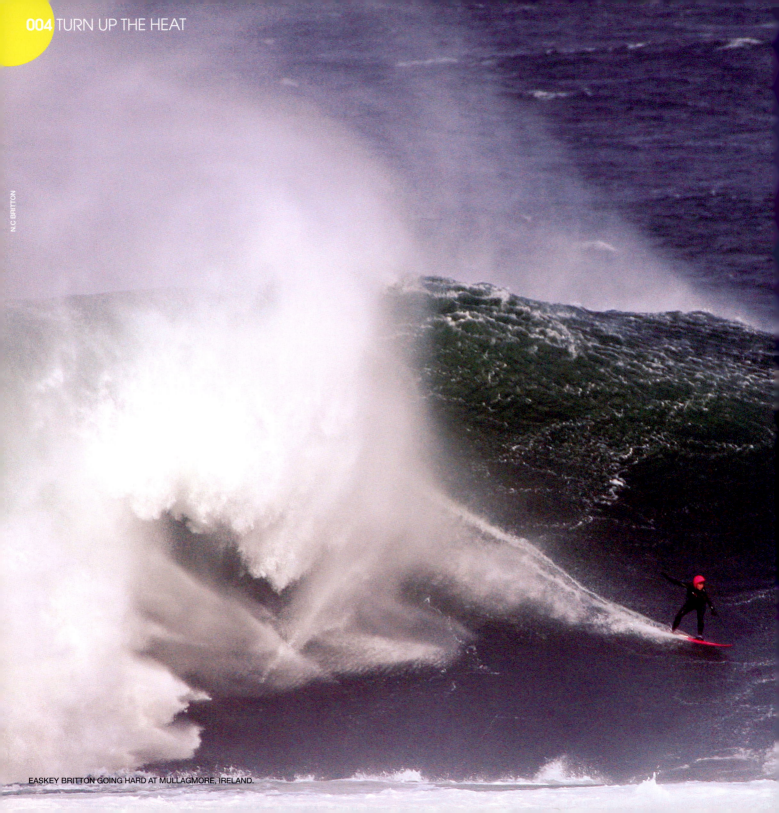

N.C BRITTON

EASKEY BRITTON GOING HARD AT MULLAGMORE, IRELAND.

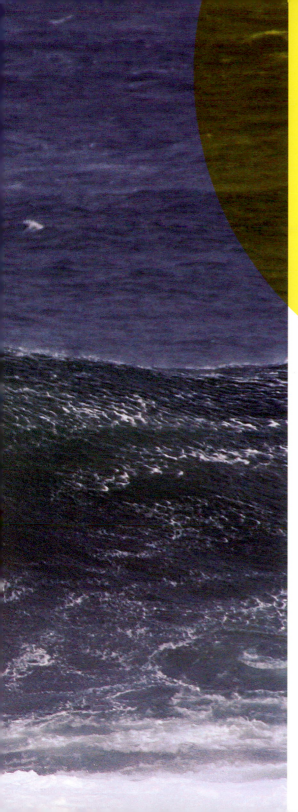

RIDING BIG WAVES

Big surf separates the women from the girls – it's pretty scary! So here's some advice for being confident in big surf with pro surfers Kirsty Jones and Easkey Britton.

BEFORE YOU GO

Before thinking about surfing big waves, make sure you've checked the swell forecast, paying particular attention to the wave period so you know it's not going to pick up dramatically while you're out. Make sure you know what the tide is doing and how it affects the spot you're surfing. Waves can turn from mellow and easy to powerful and shallow over the course of a session. Keeping your body fit and healthy will definitely help you in more challenging conditions, and will help give you the energy and stamina you need when tackling big waves.

TAKE YOUR TIME

Watch the surf for a good 10-15 minutes before you paddle out so you know what size the set waves are. That way you won't get any nasty surprises when you get out there. Better still surf with a friend who knows the break. Make sure you choose the safest place to get in and out. It's not necessarily the quickest way in. Watch other surfers getting in and out and don't be afraid to ask. Try to suss out where the best place to sit is then, when you first get out, you might want to find a spot where the waves aren't breaking so you can watch what's going on and where other people are catching them.

STAY CALM AND AWARE

Whether you want to catch the larger set waves or get away from then, you have to spot them early and that means being aware every second you're out there. Be ready to paddle hard to get further out before a set breaks or to position yourself in the right place to catch it.

The first time you see a six foot wave coming towards you, you may think it's the end of the world. But stay calm and have faith that you can cope. You will soon find out it's very calm under the wave, but you have to take the plunge and do if for the first time.

If you don't think that you can duckdive it, have a go at diving under the wave without the board. Check there is no one behind you, then bail your board and dive down under the wave a few seconds before it gets to you. Make sure you've got a good leash if you're trying this!

Your breathing affects every cell in your body. If you learn how to breathe properly, you will notice your nerves calming and your muscles relaxing, making paddling easier and your energy and awareness will increase. Practising simple breathing exercises helps to keep you calm when you go under the water, and can help increase your lung capacity

TOTAL COMMITMENT

Be sure you want the wave, because if you hesitate you're over the falls before you know it. You have to paddle hard because you really don't want to miss the wave as it could leave you in the line of fire for the rest of the set – and the impact zone isn't the nicest place to be. So set your line and go! No matter how scary the drop is you have to take off with absolute commitment.

Once you're up, stay low, keep your knees bent and expect to feel a lot of speed. A low centre of gravity helps you to control the extra speed and keep your balance, and a good bottom turn is essential. Drop right down the bottom and stay really compressed to help you harness the power of the wave. Reach out and touch the wave face to get the board right on its rail and drive off the bottom whilst eyeing up the next section down the line.

You'll probably be thinking "get me off of this thing!" but gun it for the end, and once you're there give it a big whoop and celebrate – you've just ridden your first big wave, good on you gal!

Facing your fears is the only way improve and progress to another level. Just remember to know your limits, be realistic, and sometimes be ready to acknowledge the power of the ocean and take a step back...

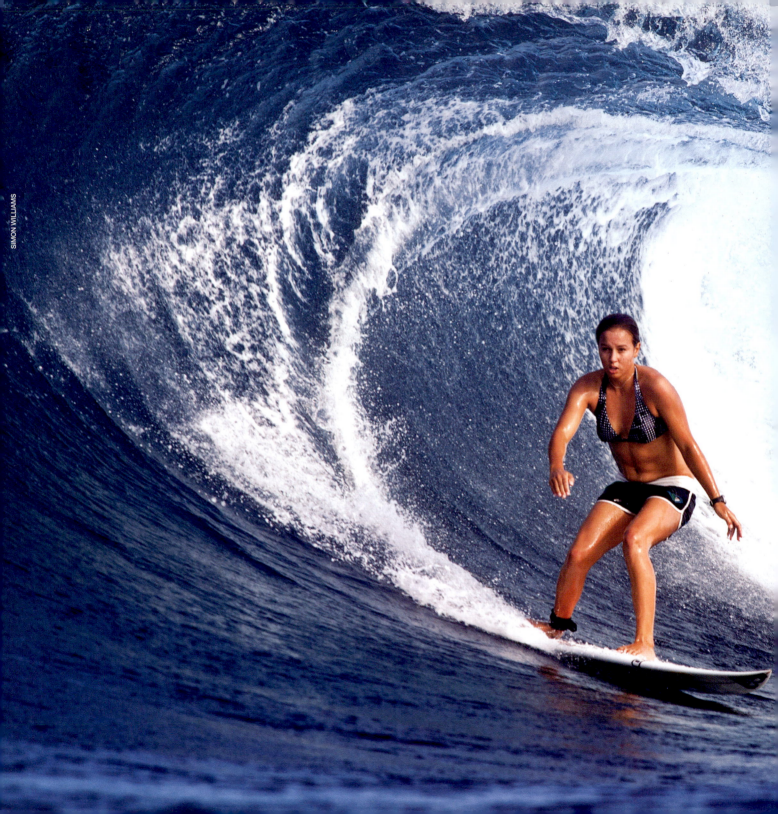

Sally Fitzgibbons

21-year-old Sally Fitzgibbons from Gerroa in Australia is a freakily talented surfer. She started surfing competitively at an early age, winning her first major contest – the ASP Pro Junior – at 16. Since then she has continued to win titles, and is being touted as one of the few contenders in a position to knock four times world champion Stephanie Gilmore off the top spot. Her path to surfing superstardom wasn't clear cut though – she was previously tipped as a long distance running champ with one eye on an Olympic medal – thankfully she chose surfboards over running shoes and everyone has been trying to keep up with her ever since.

Sally, how did you get into surfing?
I started surfing when I was six – with my dad and three older brothers teaching me and pushing me onto waves. I thought it was really cool because my brothers did it and everyone around town surfed so it was pretty natural to take it up.

What does a typical day involve?
Being a professional surfer there are so many changes in plans and uncertainties that there's rarely a typical day. Most often the day will involve – if I'm not en route to an event – surfing, training and organising the next trip away. Or sponsors trying to squeeze in a photo shoot or two.

What challenges you in the surf?
So many things challenge me, whether it's the conditions, a manoeuvre that I'm working on, or just competing against the best surfers in the world! There is always something to work on and that's why it's so addictive, it's that constant challenge.

Which surfers inspire you?
I admire so many surfers. I take bits and pieces that I like from the best surfers and try to implement it in what I'm doing. I do admire Kelly Slater and Layne Beachley as being 'greats' in our sport, and really admire their sheer drive to have achieved so much.

What's most precious thing you own?
My boards and my Lakers jersey!

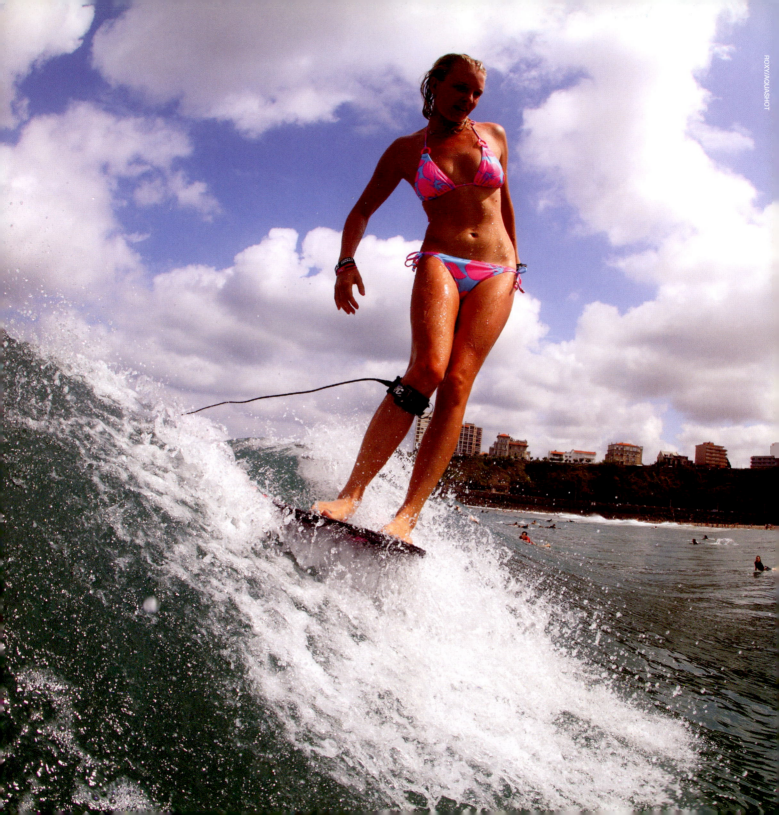

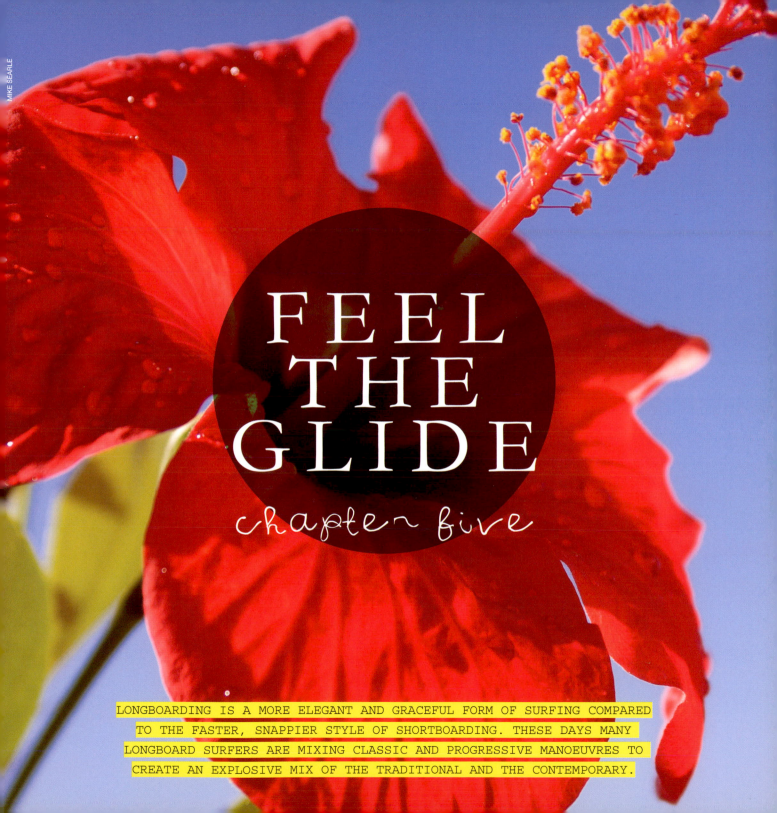

FEEL THE GLIDE

chapter five

LONGBOARDING IS A MORE ELEGANT AND GRACEFUL FORM OF SURFING COMPARED TO THE FASTER, SNAPPIER STYLE OF SHORTBOARDING. THESE DAYS MANY LONGBOARD SURFERS ARE MIXING CLASSIC AND PROGRESSIVE MANOEUVRES TO CREATE AN EXPLOSIVE MIX OF THE TRADITIONAL AND THE CONTEMPORARY.

BASIC LONGBOARD MANOEUVRES

with CANDICE O'DONNELL

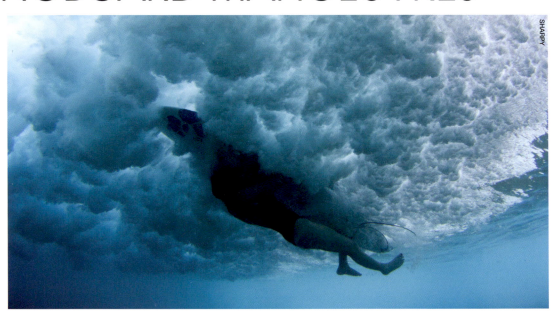

SHARPY

TURTLE ROLL

How to do the turtle roll with Brit pro longboarder Candice O'Donnell.
1. Be prepared and committed, timing is crucial coming into a roll.
2. Grasp your board on each rail, roll and hold on tightly – don't let go!
3. Drop your body down under the board once you've rolled, so it acts like an anchor.

TRIM

This is where you position the board in the fastest part of the wave and get the board achieving its maximum speed. To do this the surfer walks forward on the board to speed it up and to prevent it from stalling, then moves back towards the tail to slow the board down and stop it from nose diving. It's a balancing act!

SIMON WILLIAMS

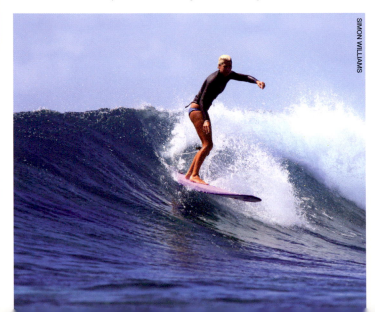

SIMON WILLIAMS

TAKEOFF

Getting the board in the best position on the wave has a lot to with the takeoff. Options include the 'fade' takeoff, to set the board up to so the tail is in the curl of the wave ready for nose riding, and the 'angle' takeoff to gain speed.

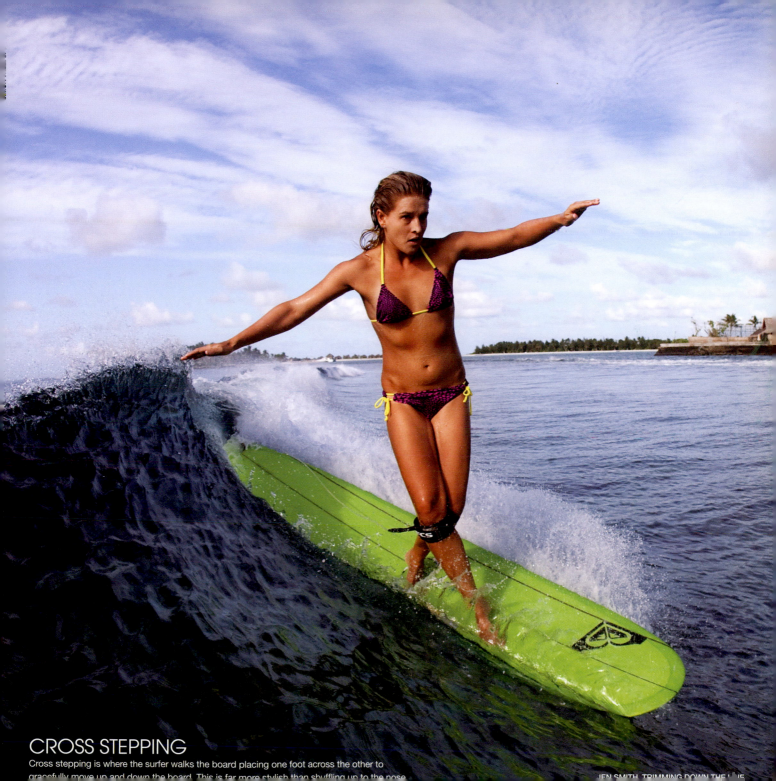

CROSS STEPPING

Cross stepping is where the surfer walks the board placing one foot across the other to gracefully move up and down the board. This is far more stylish than shuffling up to the nose.

JEN SMITH, TRIMMING DOWN THE LINE

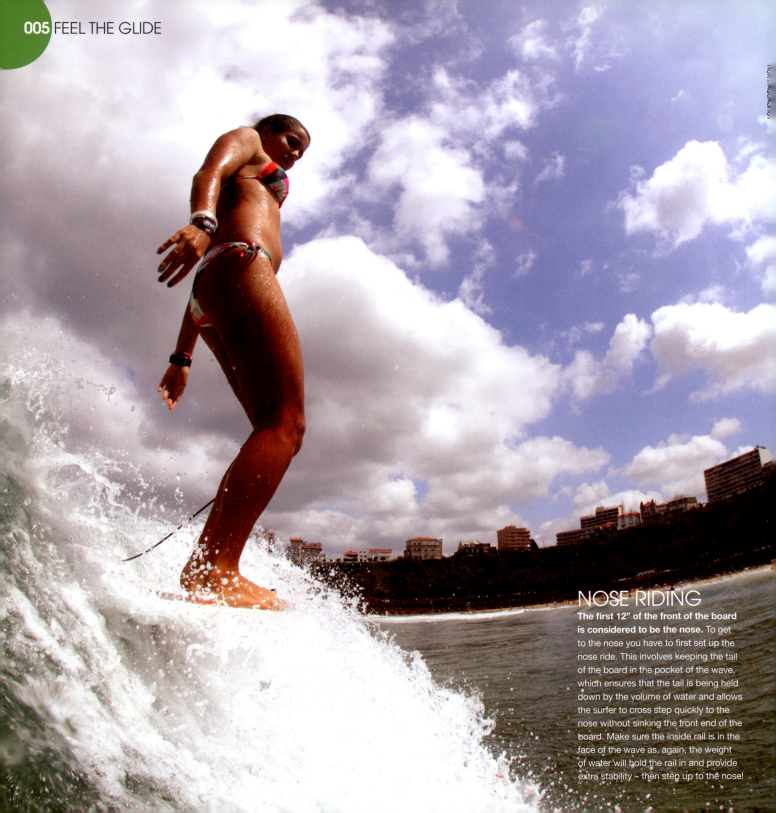

NOSE RIDING

The first 12" of the front of the board is considered to be the nose. To get to the nose you have to first set up the nose ride. This involves keeping the tail of the board in the pocket of the wave, which ensures that the tail is being held down by the volume of water and allows the surfer to cross step quickly to the nose without sinking the front end of the board. Make sure the inside rail is in the face of the wave as, again, the weight of water will hold the rail in and provide extra stability – then step up to the nose!

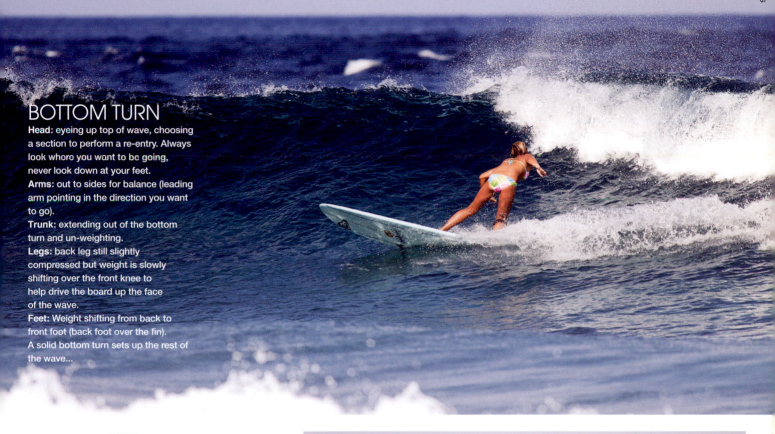

BOTTOM TURN

Head: eyeing up top of wave, choosing a section to perform a re-entry. Always look where you want to be going, never look down at your feet.

Arms: out to sides for balance (leading arm pointing in the direction you want to go).

Trunk: extending out of the bottom turn and un-weighting.

Legs: back leg still slightly compressed but weight is slowly shifting over the front knee to help drive the board up the face of the wave.

Feet: Weight shifting from back to front foot (back foot over the fin). A solid bottom turn sets up the rest of the wave...

PRO TIPS

with CANDICE O'DONNELL

TOP AND BOTTOM TURNS

Turning a longboard is a lot harder than turning a shortboard due to its length and the fact that you have more rail in the water which makes everything slower and more drawn out. A longboarder has to move towards the back of the board to enable them to manoeuvre the board around with a push from the knees and a swing of the arms in the direction of the turn. A good longboarder will make this move look effortless.

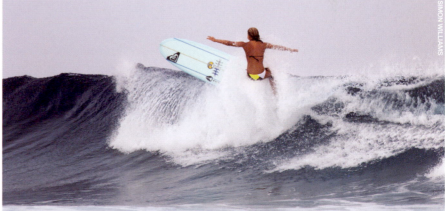

FLOATER

This requires a fair amount of speed to initially drive the board up the wave, ride along on top of the breaking wave before plunging back down onto the face of the wave or the white water if the wave has closed out.

ADVANCED MANOEUVRES

CUT BACK

A cutback can be performed when the board has raced ahead of the breaking wave onto the flat section, here the board will naturally slow down. To reposition the board, a surfer will turn the board back towards the breaking wave, putting the board back into the more powerful 'pocket' of the wave and gaining speed. The whole time a surfer is on a wave they are positioning and repositioning themselves to ensure optimum speed.

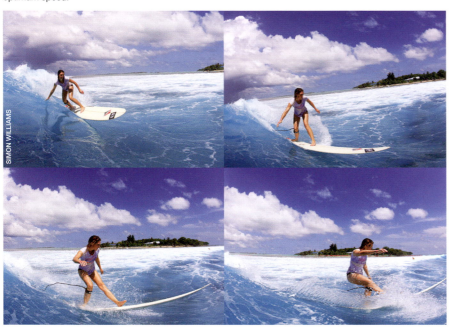

SIMON WILLIAMS

OFF THE LIP

By turning the board and heading up to the top of the wave a surfer can get a large amount of the board out of the wave before swinging it back down with the white water and continuing to trim along the wave.

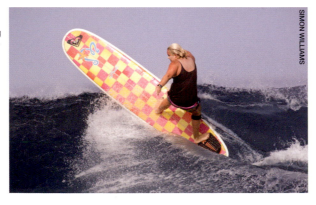

SIMON WILLIAMS

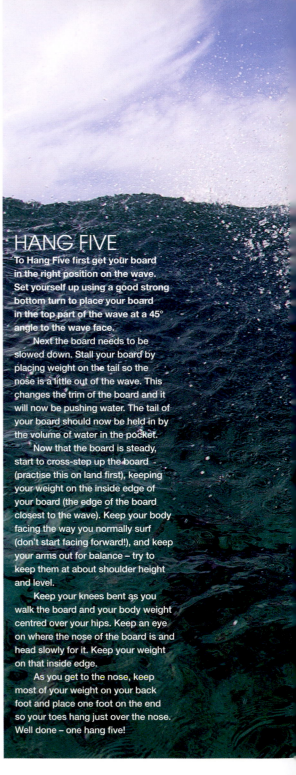

HANG FIVE

To Hang Five first get your board in the right position on the wave. Set yourself up using a good strong bottom turn to place your board in the top part of the wave at a 45° angle to the wave face.

Next the board needs to be slowed down. Stall your board by placing weight on the tail so the nose is a little out of the wave. This changes the trim of the board and it will now be pushing water. The tail of your board should now be held in by the volume of water in the pocket.

Now that the board is steady, start to cross-step up the board (practise this on land first), keeping your weight on the inside edge of your board (the edge of the board closest to the wave). Keep your body facing the way you normally surf (don't start facing forward!), and keep your arms out for balance – try to keep them at about shoulder height and level.

Keep your knees bent as you walk the board and your body weight centred over your hips. Keep an eye on where the nose of the board is and head slowly for it. Keep your weight on that inside edge.

As you get to the nose, keep most of your weight on your back foot and place one foot on the end so your toes hang just over the nose. Well done – one hang five!

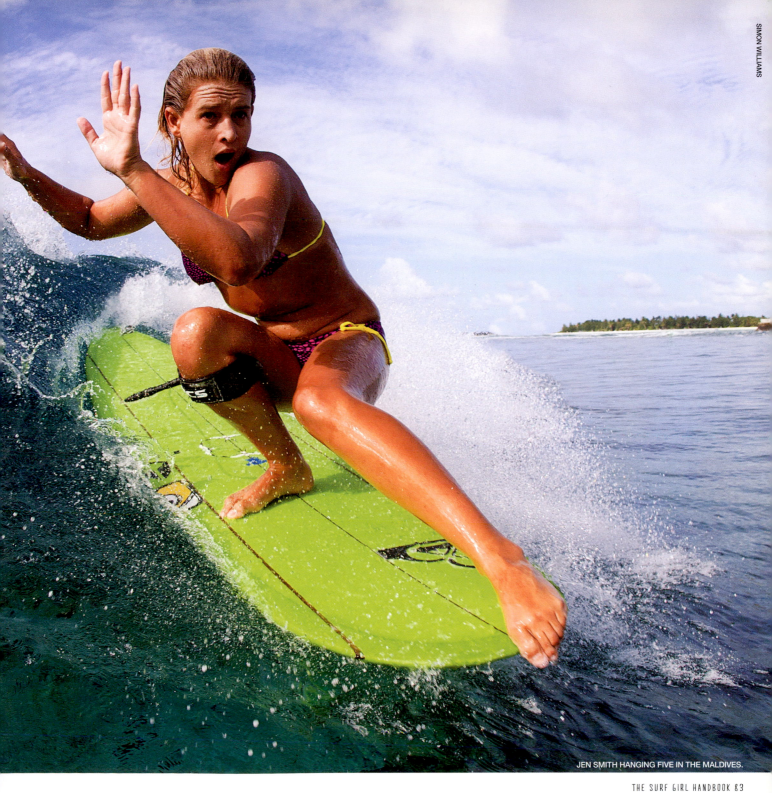

JEN SMITH HANGING FIVE IN THE MALDIVES.

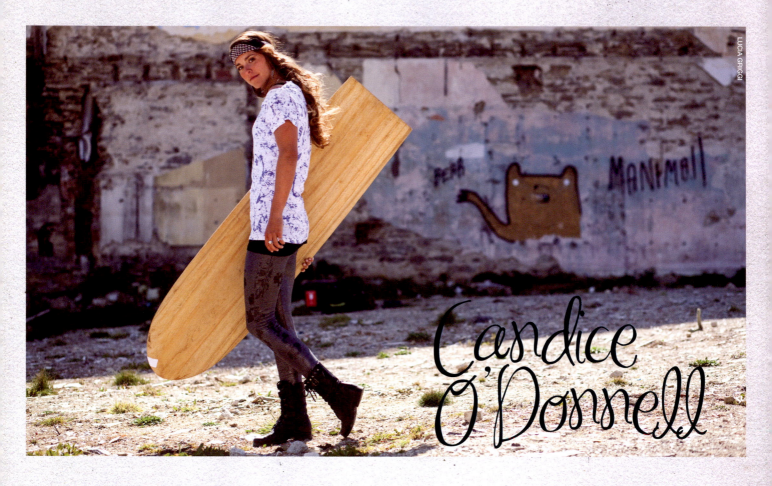

LUCIA GRIGGI

Candice O'Donnell

Candice grew up under the influence of her father, Tony, a longboard lover himself. Her journey began as a bodyboarder and surf lifesaver, and she dedicates her first longboarding days to discovering Matt Beavis' boards. Candice likes to be experimental both in and out of the ocean. She's just got an alaia (a finless wooden board) which is adding another dimension to her wave riding. Candice admits, 'It's a tricky thing to ride. Your patience will be tested, but once you've tuned in and stood up for the first time, you'll never look back. The alaia teaches you about patience, timing, speed, and elegance. It's really learning how to surf all over again!"

Aside from pushing the envelope with her surfing, Candice's passion extends to – and in fact may be more directed towards – her artistic experimentations with paints, resins and varnish. She creates a mixed-media style using her photographs as a base, and develops her painting from there. They have a very urban feel, with writing on them, and are mounted on alternative surfaces – on anything that inspires her.

She's even exhibited at the Roxy Jam in Biarritz last summer instead of competing. "I'm really excited to be stepping back from the competitive side and expressing my creativity through my art and my love of photography," she says. "Competing and training full time can become very demanding, and for every professional athlete there comes a day when they decide it's time to either stop or to slow down." This sums up Candice's attitude to surfing – a sport that, at the end of the day, is for fun and should be pursued for the pure love of it.

So, who's influenced Candice's distinct longboarding style and enabled her to achieve so much in her sport? "There are so many great female surfers out there nowadays that it's hard to say," says Candice.

"Kassia Meador has been a major influence for me, and a real asset to woman's longboarding. With her style, elegance and grace she's an inspiration, and we're always bouncing creative ideas off each other too.' Other surfers who Candice cites as having shaped her style and attitude include Lisa Anderson, Lee Ann Curran and Leah Dawson from Hawaii.

Does Candice see herself being as successful with her art or music as she has been with her surfing? "Practice makes perfect and I still have loads to learn. Whatever I'm doing I find it interesting because it is a constant learning process. I like to push myself in all areas to pursue my dreams, and to feel like I am living my life to its fullest."

So, any more projects on the pipeline, or new artistic directions planned? "I'm just going with the flow," says Candice casually. "I'll keep you posted though!"

Interview by Lucia Griggi

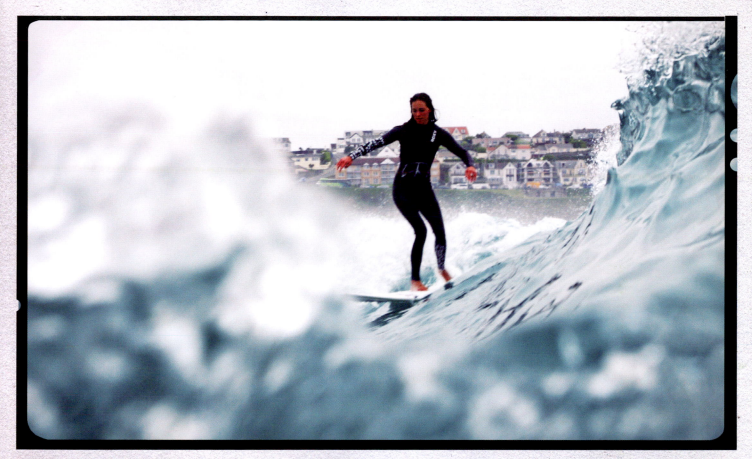

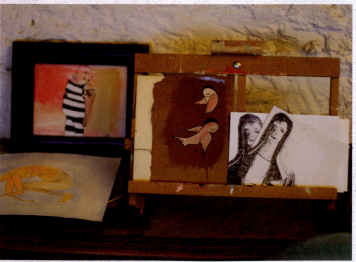

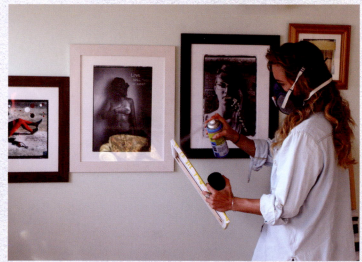

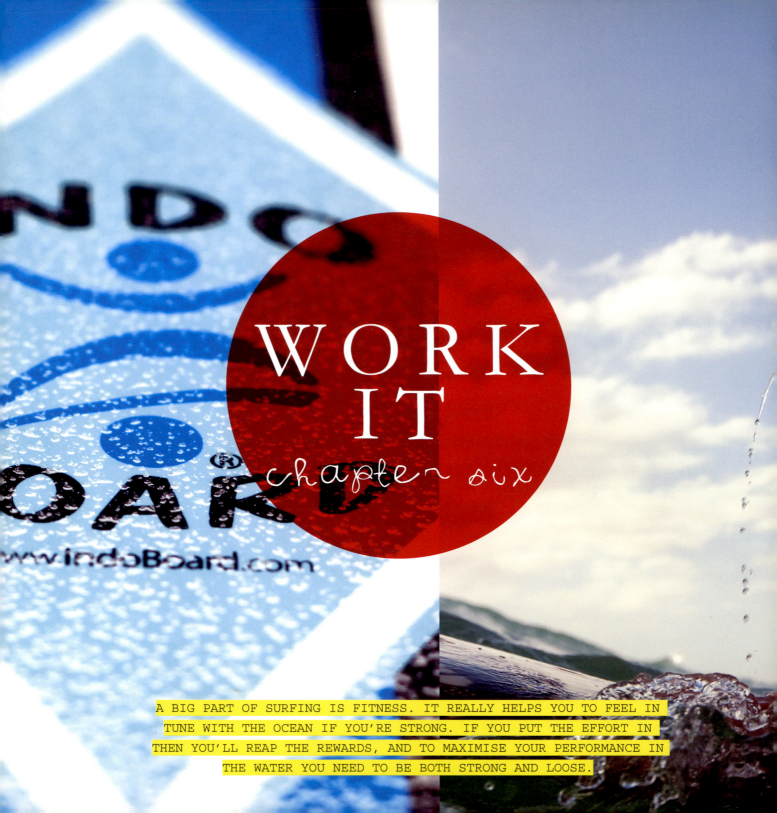

WORK IT

chapter six

A BIG PART OF SURFING IS FITNESS. IT REALLY HELPS YOU TO FEEL IN TUNE WITH THE OCEAN IF YOU'RE STRONG. IF YOU PUT THE EFFORT IN THEN YOU'LL REAP THE REWARDS, AND TO MAXIMISE YOUR PERFORMANCE IN THE WATER YOU NEED TO BE BOTH STRONG AND LOOSE.

www.indoBoard.com

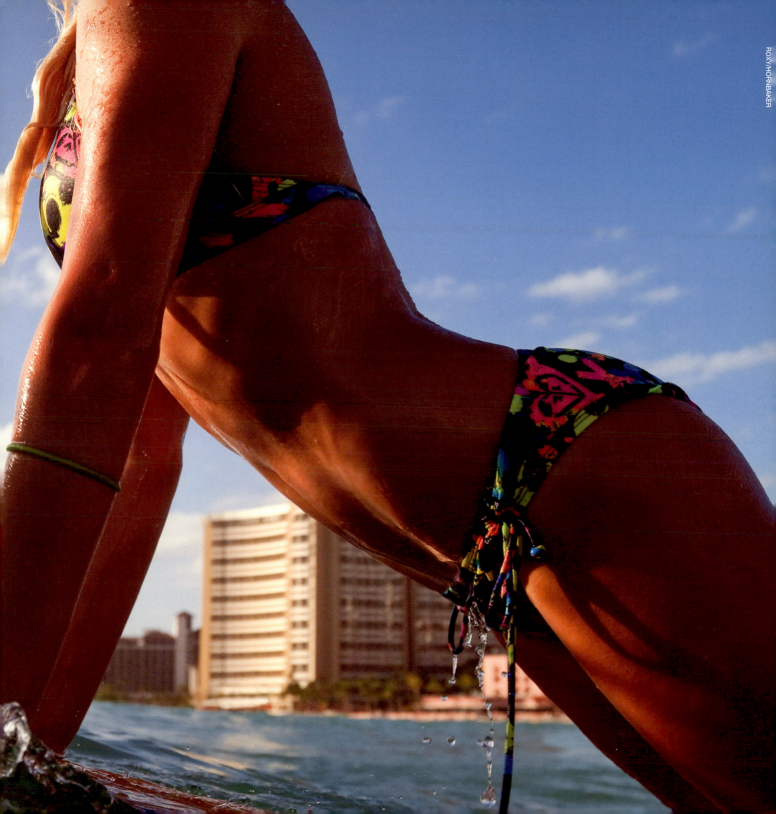

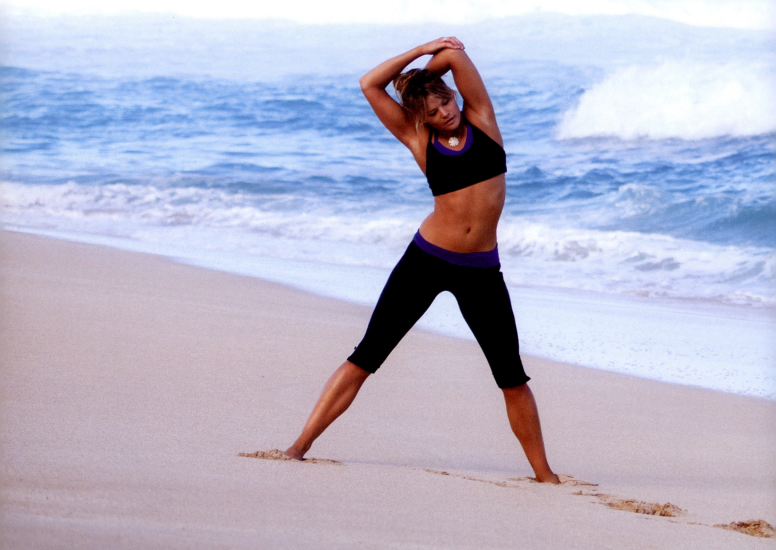

LUCIA GRIGGI

THERE ARE NO SHORTCUTS. IF YOU WANT TO GET SURF FIT, YOU HAVE TO PUT THE WORK IN.

WORK IT!

Most forms of exercise are great for building your surf stamina: anything that gets your heart rate up for any length of time will train your body, develop your cardiovascular system, and have you powering towards the next set wave.

To really boost yourself – and have you sticking in there for those three hour sessions when it's really going off – you do need to take yourself out of your comfort zone. You need to boost your capacity by continually (but gradually) increasing the time, intensity and frequency of workouts. Progression and commitment are key!

For focussed fitness improvement nothing actually beats getting in the water, but there are certain workouts that really prepare you for the stop-start and stamina requirements of surfing. Circuit training is an ideal dry land workout – through performing a series of exercises for a minute or so in a circuit based format, you can really build up your all round fitness.

Surf specific "strength and conditioning" workouts are also becoming more popular. Lots of dynamic full body exercises: pulls, pushes, squats, lunges, core and balance exercises, as well as making use of free weights, bands, pulleys and medicine balls.

For flexibility, postural correction, core strength, focus and concentration you can't beat yoga or Pilates. It's no use having the strength to pull yourself onto the wave of the day if you haven't got the stability to make the drop!

10 TIPS
FOR GETTING SURF FIT

1. Get some exercise advice from a professional – don't just dive into a training regime as you might injure yourself.
2. Stick to a well balanced programme.
3. Swim, swim, swim!
4. Improve your balance: your perfect point of balance is your perfect point of power.
5. Make sure your sessions are progressive and become harder and longer each time.
6. Use as much kit as you can – from Power Stroke bungees to gym balls – they're all there to help!
7. Always stretch after a session, and make sure you warm up properly.
8. Try to train regularly, even if the surf's good. Don't just train when there's no swell.
9. Incorporate resistance, aerobic and core work into your training programme.
10. Look at surf specific exercises that mimic surfing movements, identify those muscle groups involved and train them!

STRENGTHENING YOUR CORE
– MORE THAN JUST A FEW CRUNCHES….

So much emphasis is put on "Core Training", whether it's for general fitness, rehabilitation or sport performance. Why? Because it's your body's foundation for movement, power, stabilization and protection… So, a poor core impedes your fitness, and can leave you wide open to injury. In surfing terms, a strong core enables you to improve your power, performance and stability which will help you to both catch the wave of your life and ride it down the line with coordinated style!

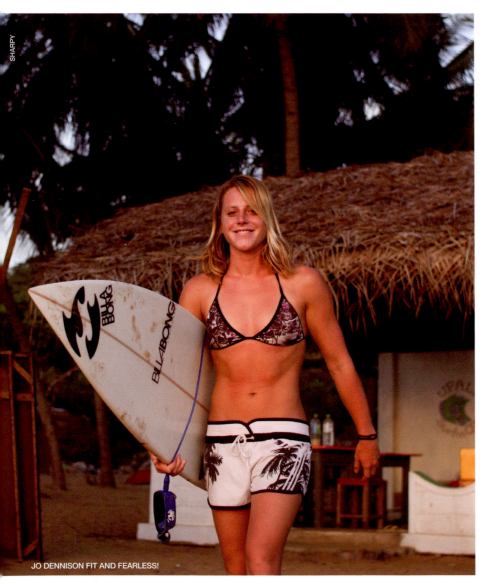

SHARPY

JO DENNISON FIT AND FEARLESS!

BIOLOGY BASICS

The core is basically your entire torso, and it provides a solid base of support for the rest of your body. If you have ever seen a diagram of the anatomy and physiology of the abdominal muscles, then you'll know that the front layer of muscle that tends to be worked to death on the gym floor plays only one part. Your midsection is very complex and consists of everything from the sternum (breast bone) down to the pubic region, this includes (if you can remember your biology lessons!): the obliques; spinal erectors; multifidus; transverse abdominals; diaphragm and pelvic floor, and it has to integrate with all of the organs and nerves from sections of the spine. Pretty complex!

Your core performs many vital functions, including supporting your spine, stabilising the rest of your body, and connecting your upper and lower body to function in an integrated fashion. It is where your centre of gravity is located. If your core isn't working, then you can't stabilise your body effectively and are far more likely to be injured – in your lower back in particular – plus you won't be able to move very efficiently. When you have good core strength and stability, the muscles in your pelvis, lower back, hips and abdomen work in harmony and will not only provide support to your spine but will improve your power, strength and performance in just about every activity you do.

And – as a bonus – working on your core will also help you develop a fine set of abs!

HARDCORE

Forget about just knocking out some basic crunches. Core strengthening is about working your muscles from the inside out, as a whole. It's your power zone! So a strong core is essential for everybody — not just 'sporty people' and pro athletes.

Going to a Pilates class is a great way to help you get started. Pilates is a perfect way to develop your core strength, and also helps you with correct breathing, posture and alignment. Alternatively, get some good advice from a qualified fitness trainer and incorporate this into your workout.

EXERCISES

These exercises will get you started and will help to get your whole system working together at the same time — and get your core ready for some serious action.

THE PLANK

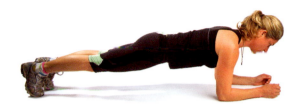

- Lie face down
- Place your elbows under your shoulders, and tuck your toes under.
- Keep your spine straight.
- Activate your core by drawing your belly button towards your spine.
- Keep your shoulders rolled back and down.
- Push up onto your elbows and toes and hold it there.
- Don't hold your breath!
- Avoid arching your back or rounding your shoulders and try to keep in perfect alignment.
- Keep the back of your neck long and your chin slightly tucked in — look at the floor.
- Keep strong in the core and don't allow your weight to shift to your shoulders.
- Hold for as long as possible.
- To make life easier... Only go to your knees to begin with.

Next steps... When the two-leg version becomes easy, try extending one leg away without letting the pelvis move in response, hold it for 5 - 20 seconds, change legs, and repeat.

SIDE PLANK

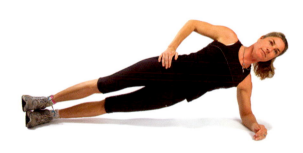

- Lie on your side.
- Place one elbow under your shoulder and keep your legs straight.
- Keep a straight line from your ear through your shoulder, hips and down to your ankle.
- Activate your core by drawing your belly button towards your spine.
- Keep your shoulders rolled back and down and away from your ears.
- Push up onto your elbow and hold it there.
- Don't hold your breath!
- Keep the back of your neck long, and look directly ahead.
- Keep strong in the core and don't allow your weight to shift to your shoulders or your hips to drop.
- Hold for as long as you can.

SWISS BALL FORWARD ROLL

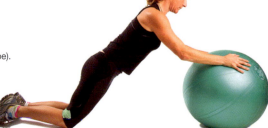

- Kneel down with a Swiss Ball in front of you.
- Place your elbows or hands on the ball.
- Keep your head in line with the rest of your spine.
- Activate your core muscles by drawing your belly button in toward your spine.
- Slowly roll out on the ball until you are fully extended (or stop when you feel yourself starting to go out of shape).
- Make sure your arms and hips move together.
- Don't hyperextend, or flex your spine.
- Roll back to the starting position, try to ensure your arms and legs finish at the same time.
- Repeat ten times.

Check out the fitness section on www.surf-fit.co.uk for a heap of core training exercises.
Stick with it and you'll start to feel the benefits pretty quickly – and you'll see your new core working for you in the water.

FAB ABS

Surfing is a great sport to get you toning the abdominals and working your core muscles, but that alone may not be enough. So if you want the best looking abs this summer, follow these guidelines.

LUCIA GRIGGI

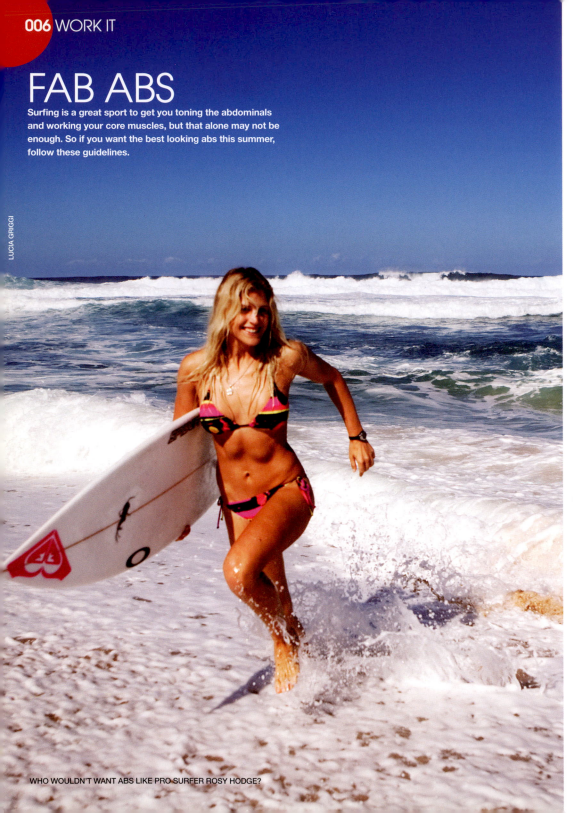

WHO WOULDN'T WANT ABS LIKE PRO SURFER ROSY HODGE?

UPPER BODY RUSSIAN TWIST

• From a sitting position roll back onto the ball so your head, shoulders and upper back are supported.
• Draw your belly button towards your spine.
• Lift hips so they are in line with knees and shoulders.
• Clasp hands and raise arms so that they point straight up.
• Rotate to one side. Do not allow your hips to drop.
• Return to the centre and repeat to other side.
• Add weight for progression.

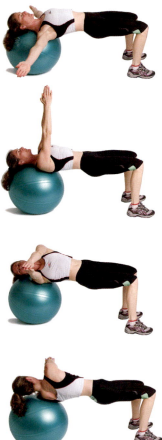

LOWER ABDOMINALS

• Lie on the ground with knees bent and feet flat on floor.
• Place your hands (palms down) under your lower back directly beneath your belly button.
• Raise both legs off floor until your thighs are perpendicular to floor.
• Exhale and draw your belly button towards your spine, rotating your tailbone towards ceiling.
• Feel the lower back against your hands.
• Now very slowly lower one leg towards the floor, keeping your pelvis static.
• If your back lifts away from your hands then stop and return to the start until you can manage to reach heel to floor.
• Slowly return and repeat with other leg.

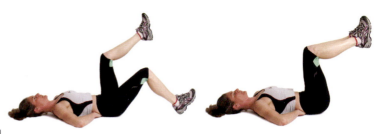

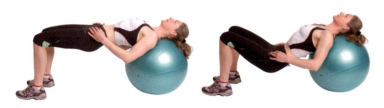

LATERAL BALL ROLL

Trains the body in all three planes of motion and is great for conditioning the postural muscles.
• From a sitting position on a Swiss Ball roll down the ball so your head and shoulders are supported by the ball.
• Lift your hips so they are in line with your shoulders and knees.
• Place your tongue on the roof of your mouth.
• Hold your body in perfect alignment (hips and arms should stay parallel to the floor).
• Shuffle your feet as you roll to one side.
• Hold for a second then return to centre.
• Repeat on the other side.
• Move only as far as you comfortably can while holding perfect alignment, even if it is only a few inches.

FORWARD BALL ROLL

Great for improving spinal stabilisation, increasing co-ordination and for activating the deep abdominal wall.
• Start kneeling in front of a Swiss Ball with your forearms just behind the top of the ball. Angle of hips and shoulders should be the same.
• Draw your belly button towards spine and hold good alignment of your back and head.
• Roll forward moving your legs and arms equally, so that the angles at shoulders and hips remain the same.
• Stop at the point just before you lose form (if your lower back sags).
• Roll out for three seconds, hold for three and return for three.

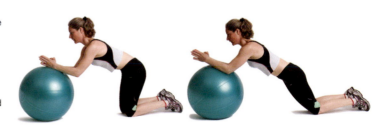

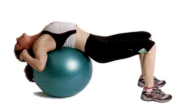

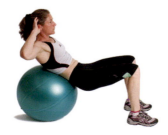

ABDOMINAL CRUNCH

• Wrap the whole spine round a suitably sized ball.
• Flex the neck to a comfortable position.
• Keep the thighs parallel to the ground and the shins vertical.
• Place your tongue on the roof of your mouth.
• Sit up, leading with the chest to as far as possible, without the ball moving.
• Don't lead with the chin, keep neck in neutral alignment.
• Belly button drawn to the spine throughout the movement.
• Hold on to a resistance band attached to an object or use weight for progression.

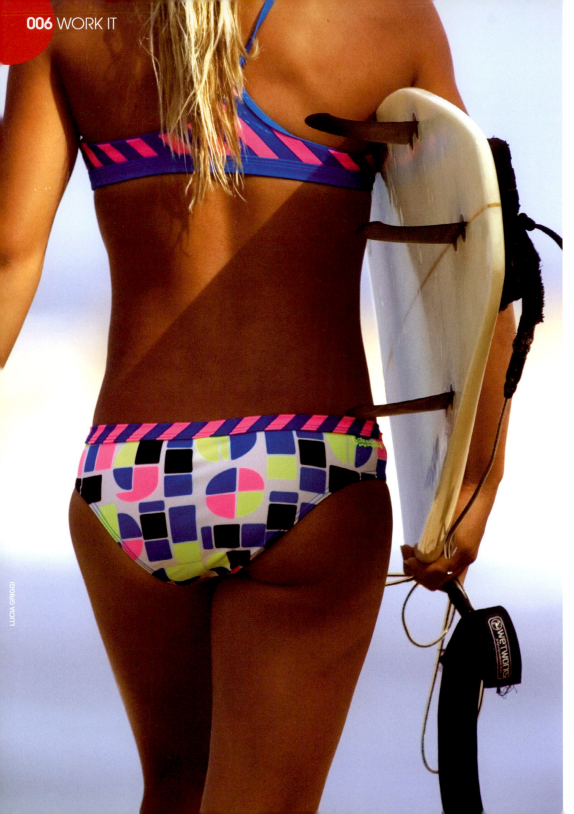

LUCIA GRIGGI

BOOTIE

Butt, bootie, bottom... call it what you like but most women want a perfect shaped bottom perched pertly on a fine pair of toned pins. Unfortunately this doesn't just happen if we're sat on our backsides all day, and most of us have to work hard to get our lower body into tiptop shape.

Fear not though, there are plenty of exercises that can help you to tone up and – providing you stick with it – you'll see and feel the difference within a few weeks.

Walking, running and cycling all help to tone up, but to really target this area and get things shaping up nicely, try these bottom-busting, leg toning exercises to kick start your programme. They'll pert up your bottom and help shape up your legs too. Plus they're great for surfing as they'll build your strength which equals more power in the surf.

So, get your butt into gear and give these exercises a blast…

Make sure you are thoroughly warmed up before beginning and aim for three sessions a week, alternating three or four exercises per workout. Workout in a circuit format where you complete every exercise once, then rest for 1-2 minutes. Then repeat the circuit again. Aim for 15 reps of each exercises building up to three circuits and gradually adding weight with each exercise.

Push yourself but know your limits – the last few reps should be difficult, but without losing form or the correct technique. If it starts getting too easy then up the weight or increase the reps, or to really up the intensity add step-ups, squats, jumps, or a short high-intensity sprint between each circuit – this will really get the heart pumping and the legs burning.

And remember to stretch thoroughly afterwards if you want to avoid buttock ache the next day!

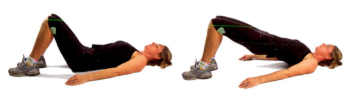
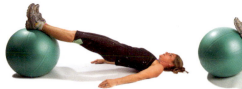
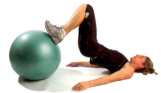

HIP LIFTS ON THE FLOOR

- Lie face up.
- Knees bent. Heels in line with your butt bones and feet facing forward.
- Take a breath in and start to tilt the pelvis back.
- Exhale and slowly peel the spine off the floor one vertebrae at a time.
- Squeeze the gluts.
- Come into a ski slope position with your knees in line with your hips and shoulders.
- Lower your back down slowly one vertebrae at a time as you inhale and repeat.
- Don't hyper extend and raise your hips too high.

HAMSTRING CURLS ON BALL

- Lie face up with your feet placed on the apex of the ball.
- Engage the core by drawing your belly button towards your spine.
- Lift your hips so your ankles are in line with hips and shoulders.
- Maintain a neutral spine.
- Roll the ball towards the body as you exhale.
- Then reverse the movement, keeping the core engaged.
- Don't lower the hips between reps.
- Always keep in good alignment throughout and keep your pelvis stable.

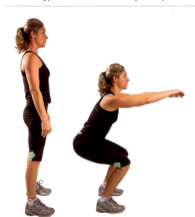

SQUATS

- Take a breath and activate the core.
- Bend at the hips and lower until the thighs are parallel to the ground (or as far as you can comfortably go).
- Keep your heels flat on the floor and your knees behind the toe line.
- Exhale as you stand up and keep your core engaged throughout.

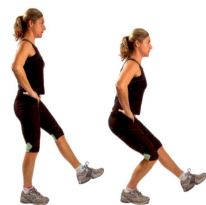

ONE LEG SQUAT

- Stand on one leg or on one leg on the side of a step.
- Take a breath and activate your core.
- Lower into a squat position
- Keep your 'standing leg' strong, heel flat on the floor and the knee behind the toe line.
- Exhale as you push back up, and keep your core engaged.
- Keep your chest lifted and good postural alignment throughout.

LUNGES

- Step forward into a lunge position.
- Engage your core.
- Ensure your feet are a hip width apart with the pelvis facing forward.
- Lower down so your hips drop vertically. Don't let your body lean forward.
- Keep the heel of the front foot flat on the floor with the knee always behind the toe line, and the heel of the back foot off the ground.
- At the bottom position there should be a 90° bend in both knees.
- Keep the hips facing forward and the shoulders even.
- Exhale as you push up.
- Maintain a neutral spine and good postural alignment throughout.

ONE LEG SQUAT ON A SWISS BALL

- Place one foot on the Swiss Ball behind you.
- Take a breath, activate the core and stabilise the pelvis.
- Lower whilst keeping the front heel flat on the floor and keeping the knee behind the toe line.
- Keep the back foot balanced on the ball.
- Exhale as you return, keeping the core activated and staying in perfect alignment.

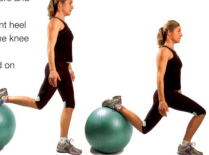

SHOULDERS

Constant paddling (unless you are conditioned), can create huge wear-and-tear on the shoulder joint, including the surrounding muscles, tendons and ligaments, potentially causing inflammation and tendonitis. Ouch!

Shoulders and chest muscles can become very tight, and the opposing muscles of the mid-back and external rotators become weak. This can cause muscular and postural imbalances. Developing a forward slumping shoulder posture is not the best look, let alone functional, and could further lead to an unstable shoulder girdle or impingement on the rotator cuff muscles (small muscles that stabilise the shoulder). Double ouch!

To paddle effectively, your upper back and shoulders work intensely and so, in keeping, your shoulders and supporting muscles must be kept flexible, strong and stable. Your body is not a machine and, whether you are out in the water every day or a seasonal surfer, you will benefit from keeping your shoulders healthy and injury free with the following easy tips.

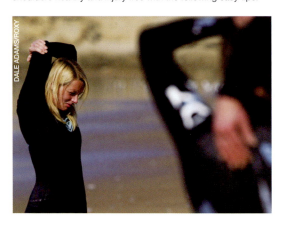

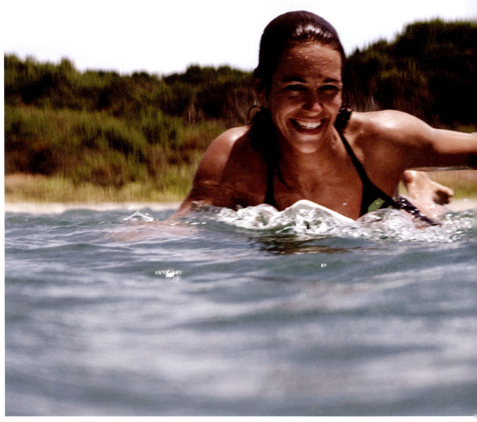

SHOULDER TIPS

An effective warm up is essential for shoulder fitness. Gradually increasing the heart rate, warming the muscles, and dynamic stretching actions that mimic your surfing/paddling moves are best. Shoulder rolls and arm circles forwards and backwards will get the shoulders in motion.

MASSAGE

Find yourself a good sports massage therapist. You'll have to endure a degree of pleasurable pain on those overworked muscles but it is well worth it.

YOGA

A no-brainer for those overworked shoulders. It can really help restore energy by nourishing and revitalising the body, as well as eliminating those imbalances and improving posture.

STRENGTH TRAINING

Strength training is important for improving shoulder performance. These muscles aren't the largest in the body, but they need to withstand the huge demands placed upon them. Strengthening and conditioning muscles will help to stabilise the shoulder.

APRÈS SURF STRETCH

Spend extra time stretching those paddling muscles – chest, back, neck, shoulders and arms – after a surf. Hold each stretch for at least 30 seconds. Using your breath to deepen the stretch should help to alleviate the tightness, soreness and aches the next day.

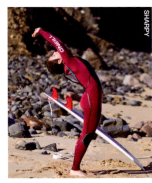

PADDLE POWER

Keeping paddle fit is tough. It's hard to simulate paddling without, well, paddling. A Power Stroke bungee gets pretty close though, and slotted into an exercise regime will increase your paddling power.

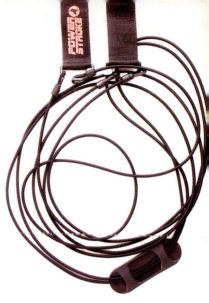

How does it work?
'Resistance bands' have been around for years and play a major role in many general fitness programmes. The beauty of them is that you can set your own agenda and push yourself as hard as you want, and you can use them pretty much anywhere.
The Power Stroke bungee targets all the major muscle groups used in upper body surf movements and in paddling: triceps, deltoids and lats. It improves muscle strength and endurance, and also develops mobility and range of movement. Having attached your bungee to something secure, there are three main exercise movements that you can have a crack at:

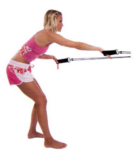

MULTI-DIRECTIONAL PADDLE
Let your elbows come out and 'push down' as you move over the stroke; imagine you're powering toward a bombie-set (but keep your movements steady!). This works the whole spectrum of paddling muscles and is the closest you'll get to paddling out in your living room. Start off with one minute sets and build up duration and intensity as you improve and become fitter.

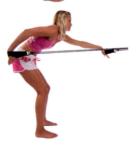

SINGLE-ARMED PADDLE
Still moving forward and back, alternate your arm movements: try to imagine you're a cross-country skier (but cooler). Again, this is great for general mobility, for strengthening your shoulder and back muscles, and also for co-ordinating your arm movements when paddling.

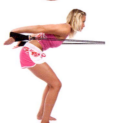

PARALLEL ARMS
Keeping your arms moving together, this is a great way to warm up and get into a rhythm. Keep your head down and move your arms through the full range of movement, from right out in front of you all the way through to behind your back. This exercise keeps your shoulder blades mobile and helps to develop your back muscles.

PADDLE TIPS

Paddling is one of the most important things for any beginner surfer to master. Paddling well ensures you are travelling at the optimum speed before you catch the wave. Not only does this help you catch the wave sooner but it also means you're less likely to float over the back of the wave, or even worse get thrown out in front with the lip! The best paddling technique is to stretch your arms as far out in front of you as they will go, one arm at a time, build up momentum then submerge your arm as deep into the water as you can, pulling the water underneath your board and aim to throw the water out behind you. Concentrate on doing big long paddles keeping your fingers closed together like an oar. Small, fast paddles will do nothing but attract sharks!

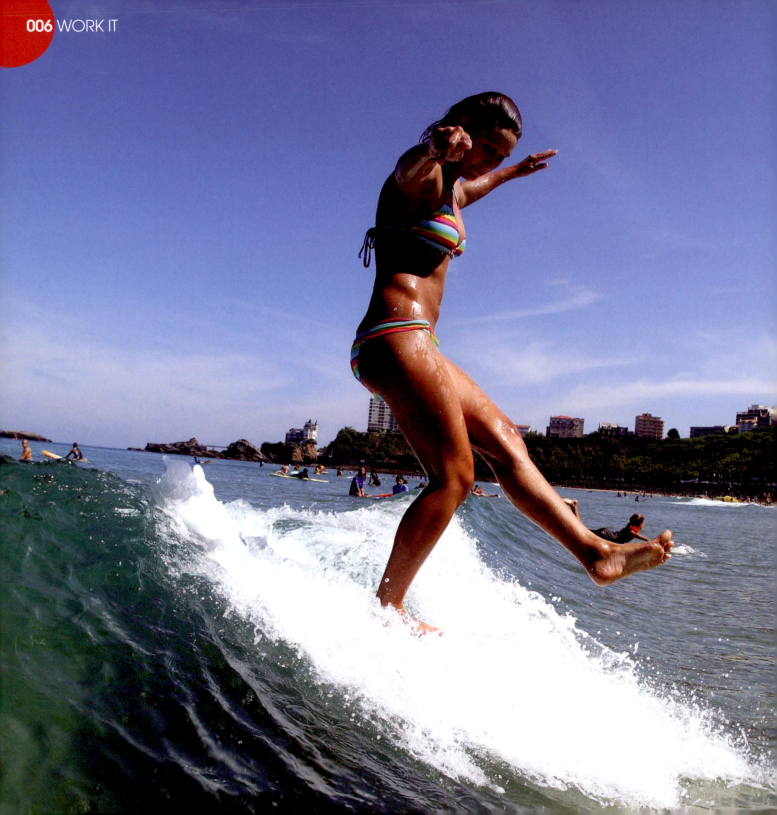

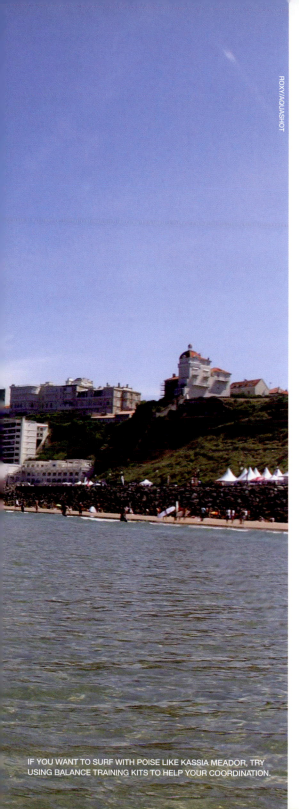

IF YOU WANT TO SURF WITH POISE LIKE KASSIA MEADOR, TRY USING BALANCE TRAINING KITS TO HELP YOUR COORDINATION.

BALANCE BOARDS

IF YOU'RE SERIOUSLY KEEN TO IMPROVE YOUR SURFING THEN THERE'S A WHOLE RANGE OF TRAINING KITS THAT WILL AID YOUR SURFING BALANCE, ROTATIONAL MOVEMENTS, STRENGTH AND MOVEMENT SKILLS.

Here are three great training aids:

THE INDO BOARD

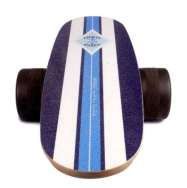

The Indo Board is the most well known surf balance tool. Used by thousands of surfers across the globe it's a very useful bit of kit for boosting your surfing strength and fitness.

You can perform single and two legged movements (such as squats and lunges), develop your core strength, upper body strength and have a lot of fun along the way.

The IndoFlo Cushion (an inflatable disc that can be used independently to boost balance and for knee and leg strength), also fits under the Indo board to allow you to perform a vast range of exercises for improving your surfing strength and power.

THE COOL BOARD

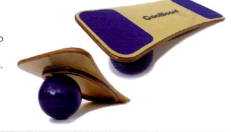

Again, the Cool Board has great benefits to the surfer and can be used to boost your movement, efficiency, strength and balance. The Cool Board comes with two balls, a smaller ball if you're new to the Cool Board and a larger ball once you get used to the movements. By floating freely on a ball, Cool Board can move and rotate in any direction – slightly more challenging than the Indo to start with but once you get used to the movement you will have a lot of fun!

THE 'BOSU' BALANCE TRAINER

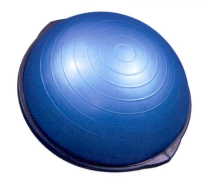

BOSU stands for 'Both Sides Utilised' and can be used for a huge range of surfing related exercises, balance training, core strength training and upper body exercises. If you're really keen on taking your surfing performance to the next level then the BOSU is a great piece of kit.

For more info on balance trainers and stacks of free advice on surfing fitness go to www.fit2surf.com.

*All balance equipment can be unstable, so warming up before any training is vital.

BOOST YOUR SURFING FITNESS
– RUNNING AND SWIMMING

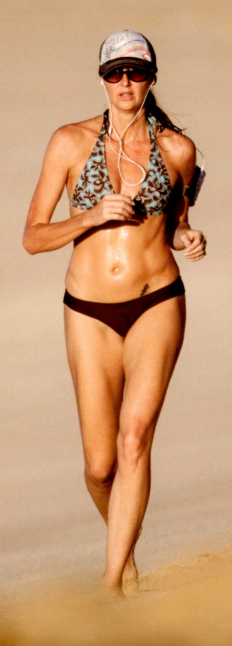

RUNNING

Although some girls run for the joy of it, most of us run because we realise the benefits. These include: efficient weight loss; increased cardiovascular health; improved bone health; improved mood and better concentration.

Although not 'surf specific', improving your fitness and stamina through running will definitely reap benefits in the water, and the other great things about running is that you can do it on your terms – whenever and wherever you want and (once you're kitted out) it doesn't cost anything!

One of the most important aspects of running is making sure you have a decent pair of running shoes. Many fitness shops now offer a "gait analysis" where they'll watch you run and determine the best kind of shoes for you. They'll also make sure you have the best shoes for the type of running you'll be doing. If you're committed to getting fit, then it's worth spending that extra bit of cash to give you the comfort and protection you need. A heart rate monitor is also worth considering if you get more serious about your running - it can help you monitor how effective your exercise program is, and help to keep you on track.

If you are committed and have a decent programme, then running enables you to really build up your fitness and stamina quickly. And it doesn't have to be boring: interval training, hill training and running outdoors is both more beneficial and more fun than a repetitive plod on the treadmill.

PLAN A PROGRAMME
If you're just starting out, then progress gradually each week through setting realistic goals.
Aim for 2–4 sessions a week, building up to at least 30 minutes of steady running at a good pace – you should be pretty knackered and ready for a plate of pasta when you're done!

Once you're at this level and comfortable with it, then you can start bringing in interval and hill training. This will boost your fitness, increase your metabolic rate and will improve your stamina and strength. Push yourself but know your limits. Always warm up, and make sure you stretch after your run: stretching your legs, hips and lower back is crucial in preventing the onset of injuries.

A TYPICAL INTERVAL TRAINING PROGRAMME WOULD BE:
• 5-10 minutes warm up: Get your heart rate up and get yourself read for action!
• 10 x sets of between 30 seconds and 2 minutes (longer sets as get fitter) running hard. Give yourself 1-2 minutes recovery between sets.
• 5-10 minutes cool down – back to a steady pace.
• Stretch...

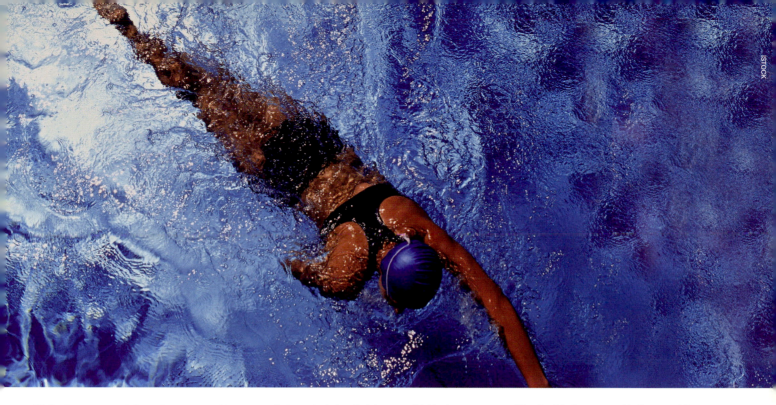

ISTOCK

SWIMMING

Swimming is the most 'like surfing' exercise around, and is a safe bet for getting you ready for that first spring session. Unfortunately a few lengths of breast-stroke once a week while you shoot the breeze with your girlfriends won't really cut it: you need to be swimming regularly and have a decent regime. Here are surf fitness coach Lee Stanbury's top tips:

THE THEORY

If you're doing it right, then the upper body movements and fitness demands that swimming place on the body are similar to surfing. Paddling requires the shoulders, back and triceps to work together and power you along – this is also the case for front crawl.

Swimming also places similar aerobic demands on the body to surfing. The steady metronomic nature of front crawl is great cardiovascular exercise, and will help you with your paddle out and with paddling around on the hunt for your next wave. It'll also help to build your lung capacity and prepare you for the less fun aspects of surfing: like wipeouts and hold downs!

As with paddling, your swimming speed is largely governed by good technique, rather than strength. Think about having a lesson or putting in a call to that water-polo playing friend to get some tips and ensure that your technique is right: more dolphin than wave-machine.

THE REGIME

If possible, you need to get to the pool 2-3 times a week (check out the cost of a monthly membership). If you already have a solid front crawl, then you'll notice the difference within a few sessions. If your crawl is weak, then mix it up with some breaststroke, and build up slowly (even just half a length at first is fine!).

Aim to have sessions of between 40-60 minutes and, although just swimming up and down is fine at first, you need to start mixing it up for maximum benefit – when is a surf session 'steady'? You paddle up and down the lineup much slower than you do when you're going for a wave, for example.

THE PROGRAMME

WARM UP: 6-8 minutes of low to mid range aerobic swimming. Try swimming 16 length of front crawl at a steady pace with 10 seconds rest after each length. Your breathing should be steady (this is usually about 60-75% of your max heart rate). If 16 lengths is too much then do less, or throw in a couple of lengths of breast stroke.

MAIN EXERCISE: 30-45 minutes. Pick up the pace.

You should take your aerobic fitness training up to high end aerobic levels, this is about 85% of your max heart rate (your max heart rate is 220 minus your age), and during this you should be breathing very heavily. Above 85% your maximum heart rate your exercise is known as "anaerobic". Exercising at around this level will take your surfing paddle power up a few notches guaranteed. A basic set of high end aerobic swimming would be 6 x100m (4 lengths) of front crawl with a rest interval of 30 seconds between sets. Again, if you're starting from scratch, then build up to this gradually: but do push yourself.

FINISH OFF: 5-10 minutes. Unfortunately that annoying rip never eases up when you need it to, and surfing often pushes you beyond your normal limits, so you need to be prepared for when you need that extra bit of power. Sprint training will push you to the edge and get you ready for when you need energy the most. Swim 8 x 25m of front crawl at 100% effort. This should get your heart right up towards 95% and leave you ready for a well earned Diet Coke when you get out!

Once you've got your swim fitness right up there, think about using a Pull Buoy (a small float that goes between the legs) to help develop upper body strength (check out Swimshop.com), or start focusing your sessions on your weaker areas (sprint or stamina for example).

EAT
RIGHT

chapter seven

TO BE ON TOP FORM AS A SURFER YOU NEED TO BE IN GOOD HEALTH.
SO YOU NEED TO BE LOOKING AT FOOD WHICH IS WHOLESOME, NATURAL,
NUTRIENT-RICH, AND WILL NOURISH YOU ON EVERY LEVEL.

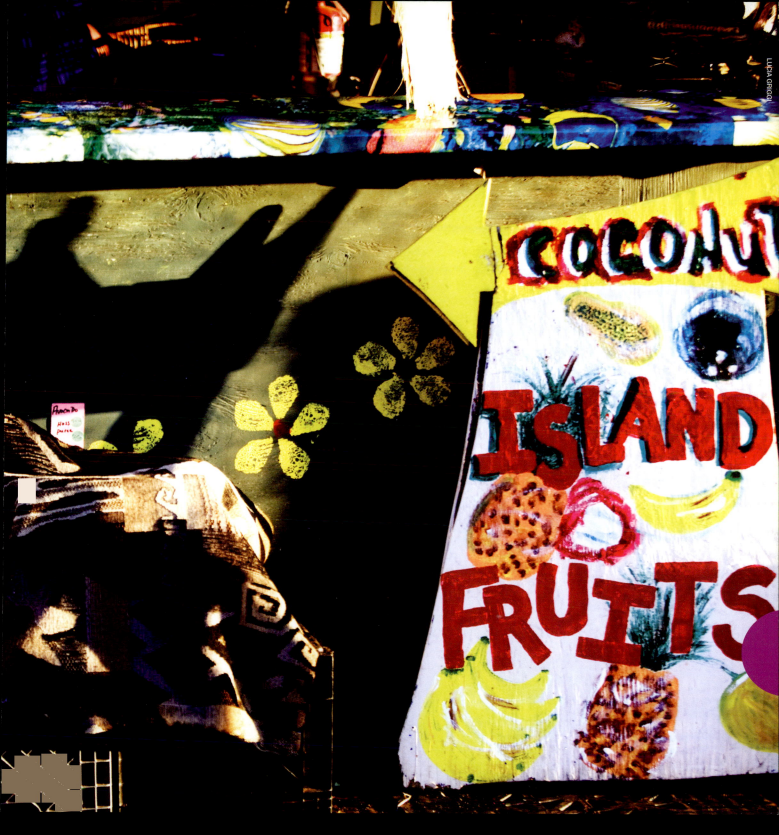

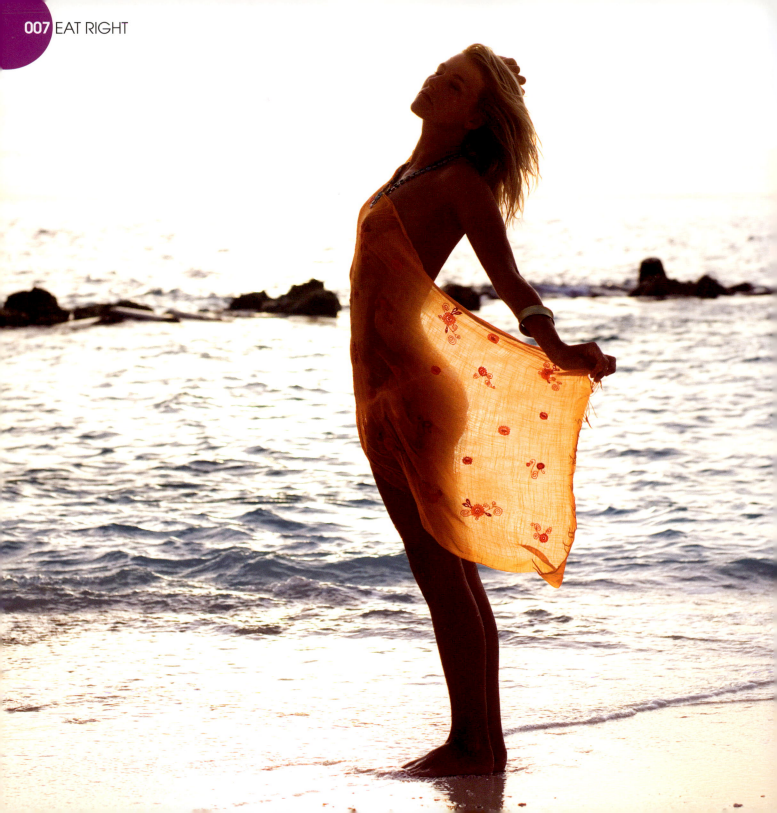

WHETHER YOU'RE MAINTAINING FITNESS OR TRAINING INTENSIVELY, IT'S IMPORTANT TO GET YOUR NUTRITIONAL BALANCE RIGHT. FUELLING YOUR BODY WILL GIVE YOU MAXIMUM ENERGY, VITALITY AND CONCENTRATION AND WILL GIVE YOUR BODY WHAT IT NEEDS TO DEVELOP THE RIGHT MUSCLES AND KEEP YOU IN TOP FORM. HERE NUTRITIONALIST PEGGY HALL LOOKS AT THE BEST WAYS TO KEEP YOUR SURF ENGINE FUELLED.

EAT WELL, SURF WELL

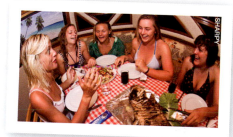

Wondering why your mates are catching more waves than you? It could be all that crap you're eating! Here's how to fill your tank with high-quality fuel so you can surf as well as you know you can.

If you've ever been enjoying a great session and then 30 minutes into it, your arms start to feel like lead or your quick pop-up is more like a slow-motion stumble, most likely you're running on empty. You may not realise it, but what you eat directly affects your performance in the water.

Think about it: you'd rather surf in the ocean than in a concrete wave tank, so why choose processed food over the real thing? The closer food is to its natural form, the better. Oatmeal (not the prepackaged kind with sugar and additives) is better than granola; wholewheat bread is better than crackers; brown rice is better than white.

You don't need a diploma in nutrition to realise that eating wholesome, natural, healthy foods will give you more energy and stamina than grabbing some quick junk food on the run. Think you don't have enough time to eat healthy? Think again! Here are some ideas for good fast food that will replenish rather deplete your energy – so you can get all the waves you deserve!

PRE-SURF BOOST

When it comes to a pre-surf meal, you want to make sure that you've got something that's easily digestible and gives you sustained energy. This will take a little trial and error on your part. Surfing after eating Mexican food is not a good idea. Ditto for doughnuts. Think about it: you want something that will give you high quality nourishment so you can surf with sustained energy.

This pre-surf meal is easy to prepare and chock-full of vitamins, minerals and fibre. It also has a perfect ratio of lean protein and healthy carbs, all delivered in about 300 calories.

PEG'S POWER GREEN SMOOTHIE

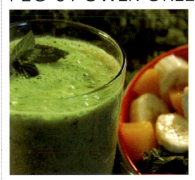

· 2 scoops rice protein powder or 1 cup plain, low-fat yoghurt
· 1 cup fruit (try frozen berries for a thicker smoothie) or 2 pieces of fruit such as banana or apple
· 2-3 leaves of romaine lettuce (for fibre, minerals and vitamins)
· 1 stalk celery or ½ cucumber (good for your blood pressure)
· 1 cup water (or less if using yoghurt)
· 2 or 3 ice cubes if desired

Blend it all up enjoy!

Some surfers (like two-time world champion Tom Carroll) prefer not eating at all before dawn patrol. This is actually a good choice if you're someone who can just get up and go without eating. But remember that this approach requires that you be very well-nourished on a regular basis. If you just had pizza and beer the night before and then get up to surf the next morning, you won't have any high-octane fuel in your tank. Instead, enjoy a satisfying meal like roasted chicken, baked potatoes and vegetables then get up and go...

TOP TIPS FOR NUTRITIONAL NIRVANA...

This is one of the most overlooked factors when it comes to flattening the abs. An improper diet will inevitably lead to a poor digestive system, which will plague you with a host of hazardous gut dysfunctions and inflammations. This is bad for the unwanted belly bulge, and your abdominals won't respond to exercise. Take heed of the following:

• Never skip meals. Eat regularly and often to keep blood sugar levels stable.
• Eliminate all foods that may cause sensitivities/intolerances for at least six months. Common ones are wheat, gluten, dairy, chocolate and soya.
• Stick to eating natural organic whole foods as much as possible.
• Avoid processed foods, hydrogenated fats and sugar. I know it's tough – but all the things we love our inner body hates.
• Rotate foods, so you do not eat the same foods within four days.
• Stay hydrated throughout the day, especially when you are surfing. Keep well hydrated with clean purified water.
• Avoid stress as much as possible as this will shut down your digestive system.
• Eat slowly in a calm environment and chew food until it liquefies.
• Limit or avoid stimulants (coffee, tea and alcohol), especially on an empty stomach.
• Drink two glasses of water 15-30 minutes before eating to aid digestion.
• Try starting your meal with raw foods such as pineapple to assist digestion.
• Drug use (medical or recreational) will inevitably lead to a toxic bowel.
• Try to stick to fresh organic or locally produced food, fresh fruit and veg, quality meats and fish – and include some nuts, seeds and whole foods in your diet.
• Limit wheat, dairy and sugar based products and go easy on the caffeine – especially if you're at the beach – it will only dehydrate you.
• Make sure you fuel at least 1-2 hours before you hit the water and immediately after. To turbo-charge your surf, try this for breckie: Porridge with added yoghurt, fruit (berries/banana) and sprinkled with nuts or seeds. What paddle out?!

NUTRITION
FUELLING UP

Getting 100% ready for your next surf requires a holistic approach. Without the right kind of food your body will never perform at its best. Have you ever tried running after a Whopper Meal?!

Don't worry about going on a strict regime – instead, mix and match your favourite foods from our suggested list to create balanced, healthy, energy-boosting meals. If you need to shed a little weight, stick to lower portion sizes, but feel free to increase the volume on the days when you've been extra active.

Three squares or six mini-meals? That's your choice. Eating small, frequent meals has been all the rage lately, but that approach doesn't fit everyone's lifestyle. Instead, focus on getting all of the recommended servings of each main nutrient group – it's up to you how to arrange them. In other words, if you like to eat a big breakfast, it's fine to have more food then – you'll just compensate for it later in the day. Or, if you prefer to snack and nibble all day because larger meals slow you down, simply spread out your daily allowance and feel free to graze all day long!

SUPER SURF SNACKS

Grab one of these balanced mini-meals for a quick, wholesome snack. Each one contains a portion of protein and healthy carbs designed to tide you over until your next sit-down healthy meal.

- Wholewheat tortilla spread with almond butter and banana slices
- Cold cooked chicken with an apple and handful of almonds
- Wholewheat pita bread with hummus, lettuce, cucumbers and olives
- Two boiled eggs and an orange
- Celery sticks spread with cream cheese and topped with raisins
- Wholewheat tortilla spread with mashed avocado, diced tomatoes, onions and coriander
- Cup of black beans and brown rice
- One cooked mashed sweet potato mixed with cottage cheese
- Smoothie made with frozen berries and non-fat yogurt
- Small handful of Surfer's Snack Mix (see next column)

SURFER'S SNACK MIX

Mix together 1/4 cup each of raw, unsalted almonds, sunflower seeds, pumpkin seeds, dried cranberries, raisins and unsweetened flaked coconut. Nibble on a small handful 30 minutes before surfing and watch your energy – and your performance – soar!

BOTTOMS UP!

Be sure to drink up to three litres of pure water every day – more if you're a coffee drinker. This will keep you hydrated so your muscles can work and you can surf better longer. Muscle cramps usually come from dehydration, so drink several ounces of water before you paddle out and more when you come back in.

REVITALISING FOODS

These include asparagus, artichokes, beets, carrots, corn, green beans, peas and peppers. Bananas, berries, figs, mangoes, pineapple and other tropical fruit are also great options and are the best when it comes to cleansing the body too.

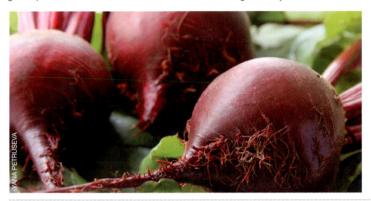

YANA PETRUSEVA

RECIPES

Revitalise yourself with clean, tasty, light food that will nourish you on every level.

BREAKFAST:
- Scrambled eggs with diced bell peppers.
- 1 piece wholemeal toast w/1 tsp butter.
- Fresh berries.

LUNCH:
- Mixed baby greens salad with grilled veggies, chopped figs and goat cheese.
- Perfect Asparagus Soup; multi-grain crackers.

DINNER:
- Grilled halibut, tuna or other wild-caught fish (or black beans for vegetarians), grilled artichoke drizzled with lemon juice and olive oil; Beet.
- Carrot and Apple Salad.

SNACKS:
- Yogurt mixed with mango slices; corn tortilla with Super Green Guacamole.
- Smoothie made with frozen pineapple and almond milk or protein powder.

PERFECT ASPARAGUS SOUP
Serves 2-4

INGREDIENTS:
2 teaspoons olive oil and butter
1 small onion, diced
1 teaspoon dried thyme or marjoram
Pinch of sea salt
1 pound of asparagus, washed, trimmed and broken into 1 inch pieces

DIRECTIONS:
In a saucepan, sauté the onion in the olive oil and butter until soft. Add the thyme or marjoram, first crushing it between your fingers to help release the flavour and aroma. Stir the herb/onion mixture for one minute. Add the asparagus and stir to coat. Pour just enough water over the veggies to cover, then simmer with the lid on for 10 minutes or until the asparagus begins to soften and is cooked through. Let it cool slightly, then puree in a blender until smooth. Add sea salt to taste – and enjoy!

Nutrition Notes: Asparagus is loaded with liver-cleansing compounds and is also high in iron and vitamins A and C.

CARROT-APPLE-BEET SALAD
Serves 2-4

INGREDIENTS:
1 apple, shredded
1 or 2 medium carrots, peeled and shredded
1 medium beet, peeled and shredded
Juice of one orange
Sprinkle of cinnamon (optional)

DIRECTIONS:
Mix everything in a glass bowl and refrigerate for about an hour to allow all of the flavours to blend.

Nutrition Notes: Apples reduce blood pressure and help to relieve a dry throat and cough. Carrots ward off cancer, nourish the skin and protect our eyesight. Beets detoxify the liver and help the body burn fat, and also make your skin glow.

SUPER GREEN GUACAMOLE
Serves 2

INGREDIENTS:
1 ripe avocado, peeled
1 tablespoon lemon juice (more or less to taste)
½ cup cooked green peas
1 garlic clove (optional)
Dash cayenne pepper (optional)
Sea salt to taste

DIRECTIONS:
Mash everything together with a fork, adding the lemon juice, garlic and spices to taste. Spread onto a tortilla (or bake the tortilla to make 'chips') and enjoy!

Nutrition Notes: Avocado is extremely high in Vitamin C for a strong immune system, fibre for healthy digestion, and Omega 3 and 6 fatty acids for beautiful skin and hair. Green peas are packed with Vitamins A and C along with a super dose of chlorophyll, nature's own energy from the sun.

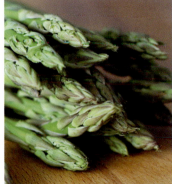

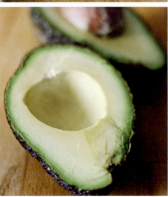

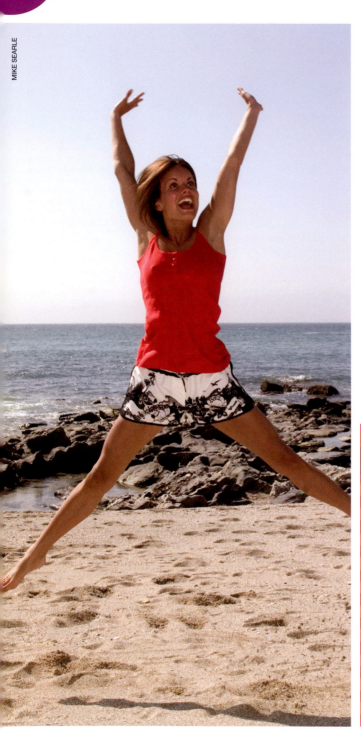

MIKE SEARLE

DO YOU NEED TO DETOX?

Detoxing is an effective method of ridding your body of internal debris and accumulated impurities. When you give your digestive system a rest from eating solid food, your body can accelerate its own healing abilities. Consider doing a gentle detox by focusing on blended fruit smoothies and vegetable soups for a few days. (Get more details at www. MyTenDayTransformation.com)

AN EFFECTIVE DETOX CAN:
- Get rid of cravings.
- Reduce cellulite.
- Eliminate puffiness and bloating.
- Shrink your waistline.
- Clear your skin.
- Prevent headaches and migraines.
- Increase your energy.
- Balance your moods and overall well-being.
- Jump-start weight loss.
- Help you to feel better all over!

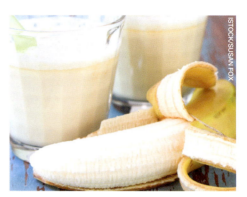

ISTOCK/SUSAN FOX

Choose the recommended servings from each nutrient group daily.

Protein	Carbs	Fats	Veggies
3-4 servings/day	*3 servings/day*	*3-5 servings/day*	*4-6 servings/day*
Chicken or turkey (3-5 ounces)	brown rice (1/2 – 1 cup)	olive oil (2 tsp)	1 cup any type
fish (4-6 ounces)	whole grain bread (1 oz)	flaxseed oil (2 tsp)	
lean beef (3 ounces)	tortilla (1 oz)	peanut butter (2 tsp)	
eggs (2 large)	crackers (1oz)	almond butter (2 tsp)	
beans (1/2 -1 cup cooked)	whole grain cereal (1 oz)	*mayonnaise (1 tsp)	
yogurt (1 cup nonfat)	sweet potato (1/2 cup)	*butter (1 tsp)	
*cheese (2 oz)	potato (4-6 oz)	*sour cream (1 tsp)	
cottage cheese (1/2 cup)	pasta (1/2 – 1 cup)	avocado (1/4 med)	
egg whites (4-6)	oatmeal (1/2-3/4cup)	nuts or seeds (1/4 cup)	
protein powder (1/4 cup)	couscous (1/2 – 1 cup)	tahini butter (2 tsp)	
* soy milk	quinoa (1/2 – 1 cup)	*parmesan cheese (1 tsp)	
*cow's milk	popcorn (2 cups)	olives (10 small)	
rice, almond, oat milk			
kefir (1 cup)	**FRUIT:**		
tofu (3-4 ounces)	2-3 servings/day		
	1 medium piece or 3/4 cup		
	*1 cup dried fruit (1/4 cup)		
	*100% fruit juice with no sugar added (8 ounces)		
	*Champagne, wine or beer (6 ounces)		
* Best to limit these items to two or three times per week			

28-DAY NUTRITION PLANNER

Follow this nutrition planner to satisfy your taste buds and keep your energy flowing.

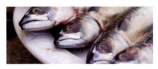

PROTEIN

(4-6 per day)

Protein builds and repairs muscle tissue and protects the nervous system.

Chicken, skinless (100g cooked)

Turkey, skinless

Fish, any variety

Canned tuna

* Lean beef

Soy meat substitute

Tofu

Eggs (2 medium)

* Cheese (60g)

Cottage cheese (125g)

Ricotta cheese (125g)

Yogurt, plain non-fat (1 cup)

Milk, no or low fat (1 cup)

Protein powder (1 serving)

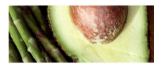

HEALTHY FATS

(1-3 per day)

Helps burn body fat; reduces cholesterol, keeps joints healthy; improves skin, hair, nails, protects the brain, prevents cancer.

** Almond butter (1 tablespoon)

** Peanut butter

Tahini butter

Avocado (1/2 small)

Nuts/seeds, raw (60g)

Olive oil (1 tablespoon)

Flaxseed oil

Wheat germ oil

**Salad dressing

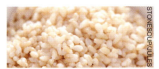

STONESOUP/JULES

GRAINS/ STARCHES

(2-4 per day)

Provides energy; strengthens the nervous system; balances moods; regulates blood pressure; excellent source of fibre.

Oatmeal (125g)

Brown rice

Whole grains

** Wholegrain bread (1 slice)

** Wholegrain cereal (125g)

** Corn tortilla

** Whole wheat tortilla

** Whole wheat pasta

** Whole rain waffle

White potato (1 small)

Sweet potato

Corn (125g cup)

Peas

Popcorn (air popped, 2 cups)

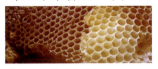

OPTIONAL

(1-3 day)

Honey, raw organic (1/2 tablespoon)

Maple syrup, organic molasses

All fruit jam

Cocoa powder

Sweetener (unlimited)

Condiments

Herbs and spices

*limit to three times per week

** read labels carefully (avoid sugars, hydrogenated oils, and additives)

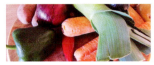

VEGETABLES

(4-10 per day)

Prevents cancer; provides fibre; lowers cholesterol; improves skin quality; strengthens immune system.

Eat a wide variety of any fresh or frozen vegetables. Serving size is 1/2 cup cooked or 1 cup raw. Lettuce, cucumber, spinach, broccoli, asparagus, leeks, celery, artichoke, courgette, green beans, tomatoes, bell peppers, onions, beets, cauliflower, onions, garlic, squash, cabbage, carrots, aubergine.

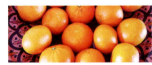

FRUITS

(2-4 day)

Excellent source of fibre and antioxidants; repairs cell tissue; strengthen immune system.

Serving sizes are 1 medium pieces; 1 cup sliced fresh fruit; or 1/4 cup dried fruit.

Bananas, apples, oranges, grapes, pears, melon, cherries, pineapple, mangoes, papayas, kiwis, persimmons, grapefruit, strawberries, blueberries, raspberries, cranberries, dates, figs, raisins.

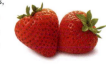

MEAL IDEAS

<mark>BREAKFAST</mark>

- Oatmeal with raisins and almonds
- Fruit smoothie with yoghurt or milk
- Scrambled eggs and English muffin
- French toasts with maple syrup
- Yoghurt with fruit and cereal
- Vegetable omelette and toast
- Cottage cheese and papaya

<mark>LUNCH OR DINNER</mark>

- Chicken taco with salsa
- Soy burger and bun with salad
- Pita stuffed with chickpeas
- Nachos
- Chicken or beef stir fry with rice
- Steak, baked potato, salad
- Pasta with meat sauce
- Chicken or veggie tortilla wraps
- Grilled fish and rice with veggies
- Tofu dog in a bun
- Turkey, sweet potato, cranberries
- Chicken salad

<mark>SNACKS</mark>

- Apple with almond butter
- Veggies with salsa
- Carrot, beet and apple salad
- Nuts and dried fruit
- Fruit with yoghurt or cottage cheese
- Popcorn and raisins
- Peanut butter and banana sandwiches

<mark>DAILY ESSENTIALS</mark>

1. Before breakfast drink a cup of hot water with juice of half a lemon to cleanse the digestive tract and strengthen the immune system.

2. During the day, drink at least eight glasses of pure water to increase fat burning, hydrate the skin, and protect the brain.

3. Before bed, take a liquid calcium-magnesium supplement to regulate blood sugar, promote bone health, protect the nervous system, and induce a restful sleep.

<mark>WEEKLY BONUS</mark>

Once a week plan for a treat. Select a reasonable portion of your favourite (less healthy!) food, and enjoy it. You've earned it!

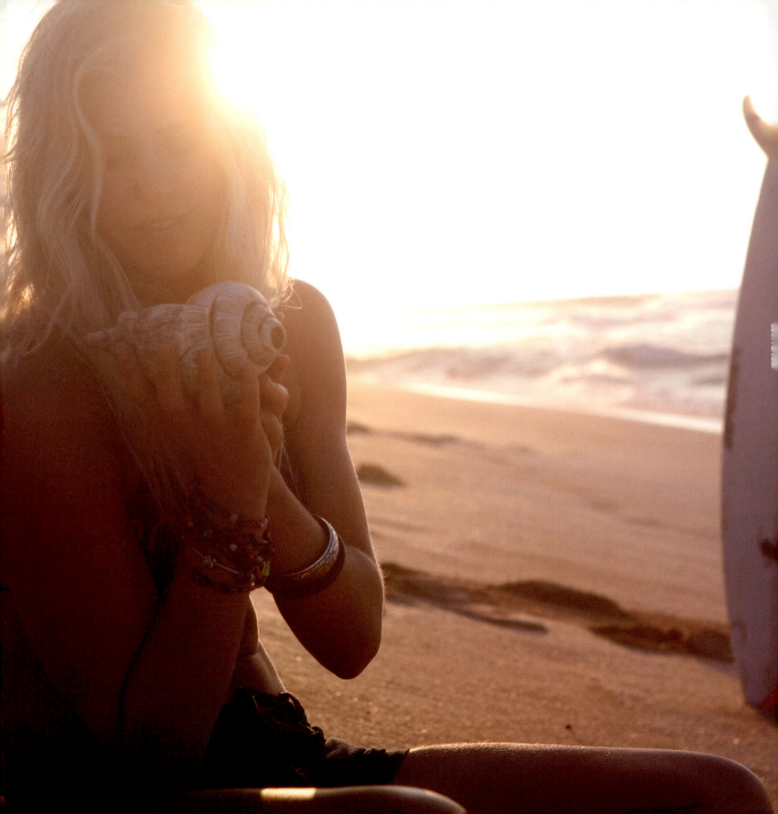

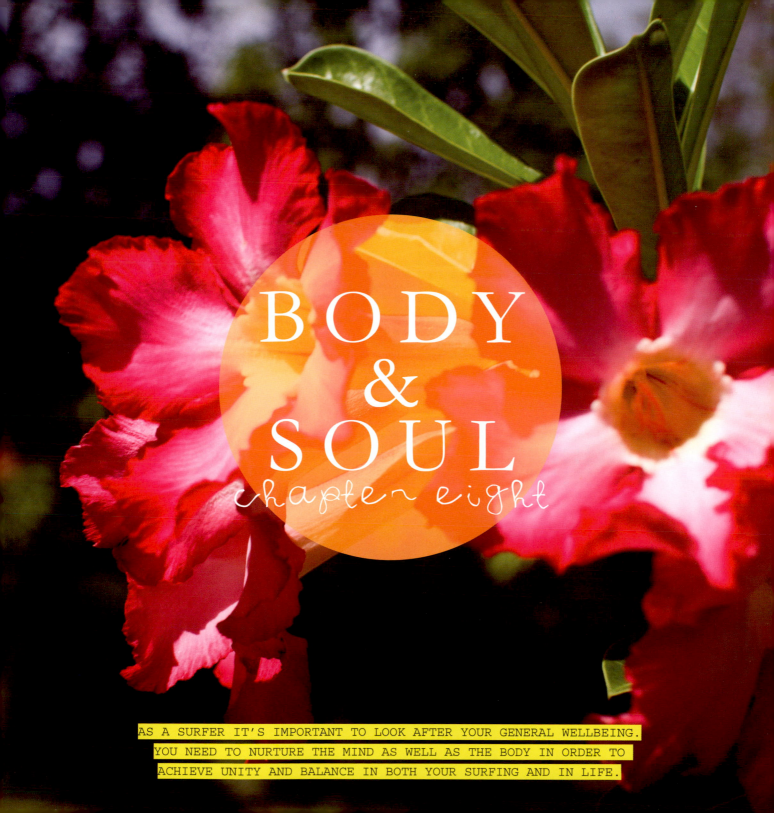

BODY & SOUL
chapter ~ eight

AS A SURFER IT'S IMPORTANT TO LOOK AFTER YOUR GENERAL WELLBEING.
YOU NEED TO NURTURE THE MIND AS WELL AS THE BODY IN ORDER TO
ACHIEVE UNITY AND BALANCE IN BOTH YOUR SURFING AND IN LIFE.

YOGA

Yoga means unity. It means bringing attention to the entire mind-body awareness and stimulates your entire body, which helps to calm and focus your mind, build your immune system and rebuild and restore muscle tissue. Through practicing yoga, you become more aware of your body, you will become more aware of your surroundings, and your flow and union with the ocean and the rhythm with the waves will sharpen.

Yoga teacher Sam McGee takes us through some yoga sequences and postures to improve your flexibility, your range of motion and strength, and to increase your lung capacity to help in bigger surf. Plus, on a mental level, yoga clears the mind of clutter and improves balance, hand-eye coordination and energy levels.

SURF FOCUSED

As a pre surf warm up it's best to do sequences that stimulate the body – we want quick muscle response for performance. Stretching and focusing on deep breathing to circulate the blood flow and bring energy and awareness to the body and mind is the best type of pre-surf practice.

When you're recovering from long sessions it is best to slow things down and take the time to unwind and breath into the muscles. Doing a basic sun salutation can cover most of these areas for focus and flexibility and going in to standing balancing poses helps to increase strength and flexibility. Going into spinal twists, flexion and extension posturing will also increase the joint mobility and restore the spinal fluid, flexibility, and integrity in the spine following your session.

SUN SALUTES

The Sun Salute is a sequence of primary yoga postures that helps to warm and tone the body, building core strength and increasing flexibility of the spine. Balancing and calming, they help to increase energy levels and invigorate the mind and body. So a great way to kick start the day!

1 PRAYER POSE

Feet apart and standing tall, exhale slowly and deeply with your hands pressed together at chest height.

2 BACK BEND

Inhale slowly and lift the chest and stretch your arms up over your head, gently dropping your head back and arching your spine from the waist. Your hips should be forward and your neck relaxed, with firm legs, knees slightly bent.

3 FORWARD BEND

Exhale, pulling in your stomach muscles and hold them in. Gently fold forwards from the waist with bent knees and a flat back, placing your fingertips in line with your toes until, eventually, your palms are flat on the floor.

4 EASY LUNGE

Inhale, looking straight ahead, chest up and a flat back. Exhale, move your right leg straight back until your right knee is on the floor and then lift your chest further.

5 EASY PLANK

Inhale again, holding your breath, and step your left leg back until both knees and toes are down on the floor. Inhale with your chest forward and your weight over your hands and toes – your hands should be directly under your shoulders. Keep your head and body in a straight line. Now exhale, gently bending your elbows and lowering your body towards the floor – don't let your chest go below elbow height.

6 COBRA (UP DOG)

Inhale and push your palms flat into the floor, extending your legs and pointing your toes, with feet open to hip distance. With your hips and stomach still touching the floor and elbows bent backwards and pressing in, lift your chest and look forwards.

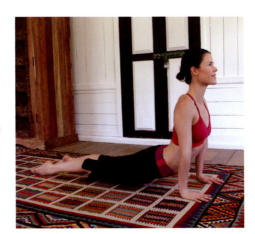

7 DOWNWARD FACING DOG

Exhale, curling your toes under with your feet hip distance apart. Now raise your hips and create an inverted 'V' shape with your body and legs. Pull in your ribs and stomach muscles to support your back, and try to gently stretch your heels down into the floor. Take 5 breaths in and out.

Note: If your heels are more than 2cm off the floor, take a wider stance. If your shoulders are stiff, open your hands more and turn the fingers slightly outwards. If your hamstrings are tight, keep your knees slightly bent.

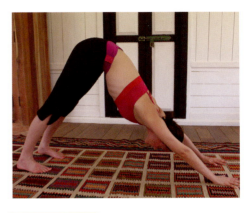

8 EASY LUNGE

Inhale and look straight ahead. Step your right leg forward, placing your foot between your hands with your left knee resting on the floor. Now lift your chest a bit more.

9 FORWARD BEND

Exhale, pulling in your stomach muscles, and step your left leg in until the toes are in line. With your feet apart, gently fold forwards, bending your knees slightly. Let your head and neck drop. Your weight should be over your toes.

10 BACK BEND

Inhale and stretch your arms up over your head and gently drop your head back, arching your spine from the waist. Your hips should be forward and your neck relaxed.

11 MOUNTAIN POSE

Exhale and bring your arm back down to your sides. Stand tall, stretching up through your body, and then relax. Be aware of how your body feels after a sequence. Repeat several times until the body feels nice and warm.

ON BALANCE

Balance in a physical sense means the combination of strength and flexibility. In general terms balance means stability and equilibrium and is very important when surfing, as you need the strength to paddle out into the waves and to get up on your board and stay there – and the flexibility of body and mind to take what the waves throw at you. So with yoga, what you learn on the mat you can take onto the board.

Simple balancing postures have many benefits: improved body strength, increased flexibility in joints and a more focused mind – teaching you to be aware of the breath and be patient. If you fall out of a balance, smile and try again. Practice takes patience and patience takes practice!

THE TREE POSE

The Tree Pose is a basic balance that works on strengthening the legs, opening the knees and hips, elongating the spine and building awareness. Once you've mastered it then there are many variations which can be developed.

1. Begin with the feet together, then bring the weight onto the left leg and firm up the left thigh muscle.
2. Lift the right foot and place the sole of the foot up against the inner left thigh, as high up into the thigh as is comfortable (but not on the knee). Feel the connection of the foot firmly against the leg to create some pressure.
3. Gently push the hips forward and the bent knee out and back; as the stomach pulls in, you will be able to stretch the spine upwards through the crown of the head. Try to keep the hips parallel with the floor.
4. Lift the hands to prayer (namaskar). From here you can work on different hand or arm variations – arms above the head or arms out to the sides.
5. When you are in the final expression of the pose, find a soft, fixed point of focus, breath slowly through the nose and be still. Release from the posture the way you went in and try it on the other side.

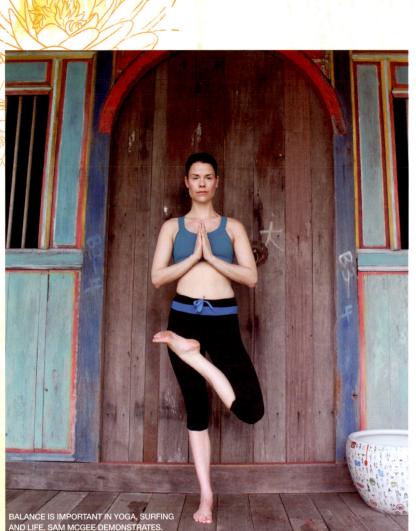

BALANCE IS IMPORTANT IN YOGA, SURFING AND LIFE. SAM MCGEE DEMONSTRATES.

SIDE PLANK

Another highly effective balance is the side plank, which works on arm, wrist, leg and abdominal strength, creating a stretch between the shoulders and arms, and improved flexibility in the neck.

1. Begin by lying on your right side, knees together and bent slightly, feet on top of each other.
2. Place the hands flat on the ground, a shoulder distance apart. The right hand should be underneath the right shoulder, fingers wide and pointing upwards away from the body. The left hand helps create stability.
3. Breathe in, pull in your stomach muscles and lift the hips off the floor as you straighten the right leg. Keep the right leg firm and try to straighten the left leg, so the left foot rest above the right foot.
4. With the body stable, lift the left hand up to the sky, shoulders directly on top of each other and look up to the left hand. Continue to stretch through the shoulders and down the side of the body. Hold the posture and breathe comfortably for a few seconds.
5. Release the way you went in and slowly turn over and try the posture on the left side.

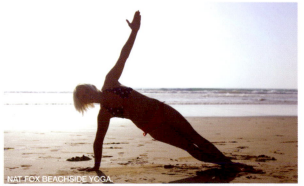

NAT FOX BEACHSIDE YOGA.

PILATES POWER

IT'S ALL ABOUT BALANCE THESE DAYS. PILATES INSTRUCTOR **AMY SWANSON** TAKES US THROUGH SOME EXERCISES WHICH COMBINE MENTAL AND PHYSICAL FITNESS.

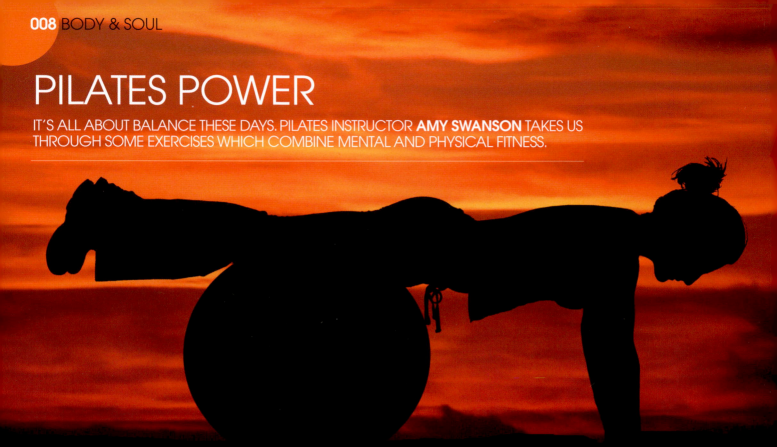

What is Pilates?

Put simply, Pilates is a form of body conditioning that brings your body to the height of physical fitness and brings your mind with it. Using a series of challenging moves you will rotate, flex, bend and extend your body and spine to gain dexterity, balance, control, stamina and strength. All exercises require a deep level of concentration and should be performed with precision and control, thus achieving total mind/body integration.

How will Pilates benefit your surfing?

Pilates can support, improve and enhance your surfing in many ways. Surfing is an essentially poorly balanced sport, with lots of time spent on your front looking up, putting pressure on your lower back and always popping up to one side (goofy or regular). Because Pilates is about muscle balance, exercise sequences will always be devised to make sure you move your body over all planes of movement to counterbalance any one-sided work. For example, it's important to do lots of abdominal exercises with the spine flexed forwards to redress all the time spent with your spine extended backwards when you are paddling your board. Core stability is a phrase often bandied about, but is of particular importance in surfing – Pilates also helps here as lots of the postures and moves involve reducing your points of contact with the floor: we de-stabilise to stabilise!

How long before I see the results?

"In 10 sessions you'll feel the difference, in 20 sessions you'll see the difference and in

30 sessions… You'll have a whole new body." – Joseph H. Pilates

However, as much as the above is true, Pilates is like anything else: you only get out what you put in. If you attend 30 Pilates sessions at the rate of one a month, the method won't have the same potency. If you practice every other day then you will see amazing results. Pilates is an education for your body and mind so is best learned on a one-to-one basis in the initial stages. Most good Pilates teachers will keep their group classes small (no more than 12) to ensure you get the most from their teaching.

Top tips

• If you are attending a weekly class, try to practice at home a few times during the week. Your body will learn faster and you'll see improvements more quickly.
• When performing Pilates moves, keep scanning your body for any unwanted tension. If you are working your abs and your glutes there is no need to tense up your face or your toes!
• Breathe! You can use your breath to help you: inhale when you need to hold a posture or need extra stability and use your exhalation to really power movement of the spine or limbs.

Keep yourself surf-fit by mastering the following Pilates exercises. Each exercise should be performed with precision and control – make sure your abdominals are scooped and hollowed as you breathe deeply and concentrate. Pilates can help to improve balance, core stability and general fitness, transforming you into a wave catching machine!

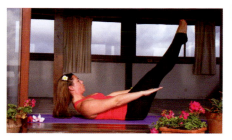

STAMINA: THE 100

Lie on your back with your legs folded over the body and connected into a table top position. Curl up off the mat and lift your arms a few inches. Extend the legs away on a high diagonal. Keep the inner thighs connected throughout.
• Begin to breathe in and pump the arms as a rigid lever up and down for 5 beats. Exhale and continue to beat the arms for 5. Keep pumping the arms as you breathe in for 5 and out for 5.
Complete 10 full breaths thus pumping the arms 100 times – hence the name!
• If your neck is sore, take your hands and clasp them behind your head so as not to strain your neck.
• If the weight of your legs starts to pull into your lower back; bring the legs back to the table top position in (fig. 1)

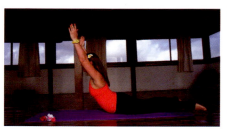

FLEXIBILITY: SWAN DIVE

• Lie on your front with your legs apart and turned out and your hands by the side of your face. Peel your spine up one bone at a time until your arms are completely straight. Keep the neck long and the collar bones open.
• Breathe in and maintain the arc of the spine as you sweep the arms forward and rock down the front of your body. Keeping the shape of the arms, spine and legs will mean the legs lift off the mat. Continue rocking forward and back maintaining the arc.
• Keep your tummy and your ribs pulled in to avoid over working the lower back.

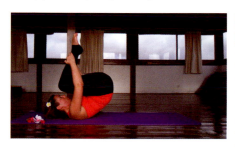

MUSCLE BALANCE: ROLLING LIKE A BALL

• Sit at the front of your mat, curl yourself into a ball shape and take your feet off the floor. Tuck your tailbone underneath you to create a full curve of your spine and balance there.
• Breathe in and roll back to the tip of your shoulders and try not to lose your ball shape.
• Breathe out and roll back up to balance at the top. Don't put your feet down!

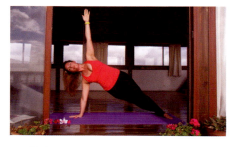

CORE STABILITY AND TOTAL BODY INTEGRATION: SIDE TWIST

• Lie on your side with your left leg bent upright. Hook the left foot over the right and place your right hand on the floor a little way from the body. Then breathe in and press into your feet and hand to lift the body off the mat creating a diagonal line. The inner thighs are connected and the legs straight. (If you can't straighten the legs, come down and move the feet a bit further away) Lift the left arm up to the ceiling.
• Breathe out and thread the left arm underneath the right, rotating your ribcage around your spine.
• Breathe in and return back to the upright position in fig 2. Repeat 3 times on each side.

OPEN LEG ROCKER

Benefits include improved balance and control, a strengthening of the deep abdominals and lengthened hamstrings.

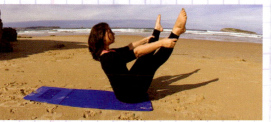

EXERCISE PHOTOS: LUCIA GRIGGI
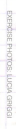

1 Sit at the front of your mat with the legs straight and the hands holding the ankles in a 'v' position. Balance on your sitting bones and pull your navel deeply in towards the spine.

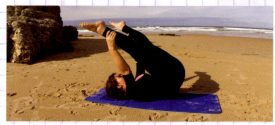

2 Breathe in and start the movement, deepening your abdominal scoop and tucking your tailbone underneath you. Drop your eye line and nod the head to roll back smoothly through the spine. Only roll back to the tips of the shoulder blades, do not let the head touch the floor.

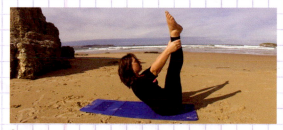

3 Breathing out, maintain the position of the arms and roll back through the spine to the start position.

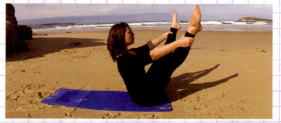

4 Balance at the top for a millisecond before repeating the movement eight times.

LOOKING GOOD

BE SMART AT THE BEACH AND STAY BEAUTIFUL FOR LONGER…

SUN AWARENESS

Ahh sunshine, how much we love it! Unfortunately what looks like a healthy tan today will show up as wrinkles and colouration spots in years to come if you don't look after yourself.

How you look after yourself in the sun is vital, especially if you're out in it all day. Excessive exposure can take its toll on your body. But you can still get that dreamy summer look (and some lovely vitamin D), if you make sure you're gently sun-kissed, and not sun-snogged!

• Build your tan slowly. If the swell is fantastic the first day you arrive and it's 90° in the shade, try and resist until the sun is past its peak.
• Apply sunscreen 20 minutes before going out, to allow absorption.
• Be generous with the cream – a thin cover will diminish your protection. And reapply after swimming.
• Expose your skin in small doses and apply high factor sunscreen every one to two hours.
• Don't forget your nose, hands and ears or the backs of knees and soles of the feet if you are face down.
• When you're in the water, go for a high protection waterproof organic based lotion such as Prosport 44 which offers protection for eight hours, or Island Tribe SPF 40 clear gel sunscreen for waterproof all-day protection.

• Use factor 30 for chest and face and 15 for the rest of your body.
• Use a PABA-free sunscreen, this chemical can cause irritation and stain clothing.
• Pile on the moisturiser afterwards. Aloe vera aftersun products really do help to soothe overheated skin.
• Some essential oils are damaging in the sun.
• Use a product on your forehead that won't drip into your eyes and be a pain whilst you're surfing or sweating. Sticks are more wax based, so are heavier and don't tend to run. Some (like ProSport) won't stick to sand either
• Get checked over at the docs If you've had a lot of sun exposure over the years – early detection of a melanoma may save your life.
• Cloudy skies can still let in 80% of UV rays, so you need to be careful even when the sun isn't seducing you directly. Hide your hide under tightly woven fabrics that don't let those rays through.
• A hat won't just look good it will protect your scalp and your hair.
• Polarised sunglasses are a must, unless you want a constant squint and diminishing eyesight. Plus there are so many cool styles that it's great they count as an 'essential' purchase.
• Cover up if you're out between 11am and 3pm. You'll never catch a supermodel sunbathing then. If you're surfing without a wetsuit at those times, consider a rash vest and shorts. (This will also help protect you from the where's-my-bikini-panic after wiping out!)

TOP TIPS

To get your body ready for the beach, revitalise your skin with an exfoliator like a sea salt scrub. Use it twice a week to slough away dead cells that can make the skin look dull. Gently massage the scrub into dry skin in upward, circular movements. Massage onto damp skin in sensitive areas such as the chest.

After exfoliating, moisturise the skin using a body butter. Then finish off with baby oil – to give your body a sheen.

HAIR CARE

You wouldn't go out in the blazing hot sunshine without applying sun cream, so don't head out without preparing your hair:
• Get your hair trimmed regularly. Split ends get more frazzled in the sun.
• Use a good moisturising leave-in conditioning spray to keep hair hydrated and prevent it splitting in the heat.
• Pull your hair into an unfussy ponytail, simple chignon or relaxed bun to keep it looking good all day. Best of all wear a hat when you're not in the water.
• After a day at the beach lather your hair with an intensive hair repair treatment to prevent frazzled, frizzy ends.

LOOK AFTER YOURSELF THE NATURAL WAY

Complementary medicine and health products are becoming more and more popular and will help keep you fit and healthy the natural way. Here are some useful products which are produced without harming animals or the environment and complement a well-sorted first aid kit and washbag.

ACHES AND BRUISES

Hemp Balm is natural deep heat for sore and tired muscles. It smells better than conventional Deep-Heat too. If you've taken a bash and don't want an ugly bruise to form, then Arnica cream is your best friend. Rub it in straight after you come out of the water, before a bruise has time to form (don't put on broken skin).

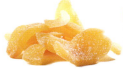

TRAVEL SICKNESS

Chew crystallised ginger or try Nelson's homeopathic Travella pills.

CUTS AND INFECTED WOUNDS

Try Tea Tree oil for cuts, rashes, burns and blisters. It's great to clean cuts and infected wounds from reefs, and helps heal skin by encouraging the formation of scar tissue. It's a tiny but potent concentrated bottle, the size of a lipstick and will last ages. It's even good for acne, athlete's foot and is effective against cystitis and thrush and fighting colds and flu (don't swallow it though!).

OVERDONE IT?

If you've had a heavy boozy night or indulged in too much strange, rich, fatty, spicy foods or coffee and have only just lived to tell the tale and, God forbid, next day you can't even face the surf, then Nux Vom homeopathic pill may help you get on with your day. If you needed to puke, it will help you clear it all out! Also useful for constipation, diarrhoea and heavy menstrual bleeding.

DIARRHOEA

Alternative preparations are not designed to stop diarrhoea. If your body is trying to get rid of something in your guts at top speed, the theory is to get rid of it, then rebuild your gut flora and immune system.

EARS AND EYES

These are much neglected areas. If you wear contact lenses, use daily disposables so that pollutants in the sea don't get a chance to grow bacteria on them that can transfer to your cornea and threaten your eyesight. For general eye soreness, try Euphrasia Eye Tincture. If you don't want to get surfer's ear (a bony growth in your ear canal) then use ear plugs, or put Blue-Tac in your ears – roll it up into a small mushroom shape first. Earplugs can save your ears from surfer's ear during the day, and your nerves from being deprived of sleep if walls are paper-thin at night!

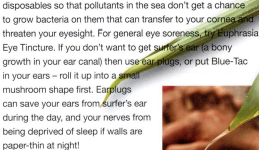

INSECT STINGS

Nelson's Pyrethrum Spray is very portable and relieves the itch and discomfort of a bite or sting. Wearing Citronella or lavender oil, however, may help put the mozzies off biting you in the first place...

SKIN/HAIR

Martha Hill Deep Moisturising Conditioner with seaweed complex for dry and stressed hair and their Evening Primrose and Lavender Body Oil counteracts the drying effects of sun and salt water.

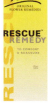

GENERAL HELP

A few drops of Bach's Rescue Remedy on the tongue are helpful after any kind of shock, accident or emotional trauma. If you've been half-drowned, got whiplash from a hair-raising coach journey, chased by a raging bull or been chucked by your boyfriend, then let its magic go to work.

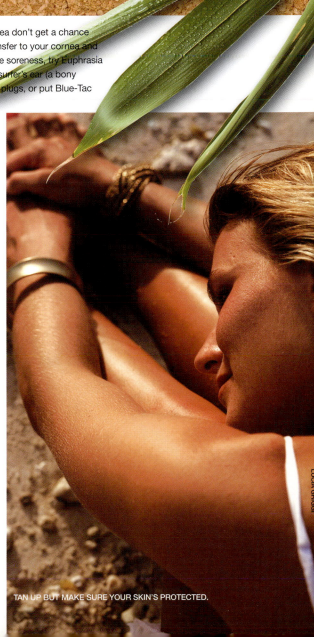

TAN UP BUT MAKE SURE YOUR SKIN'S PROTECTED.

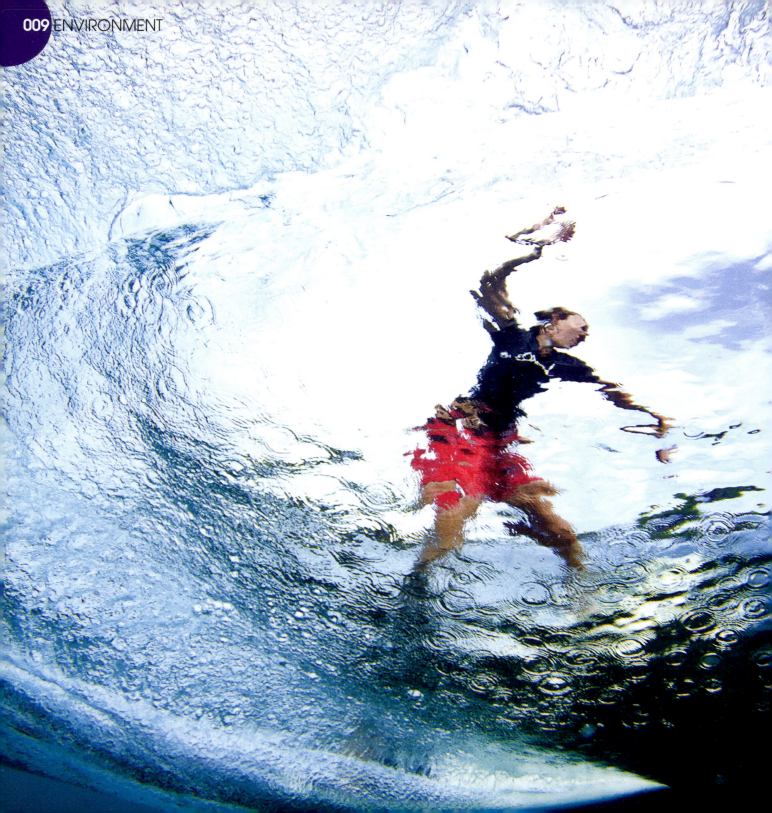

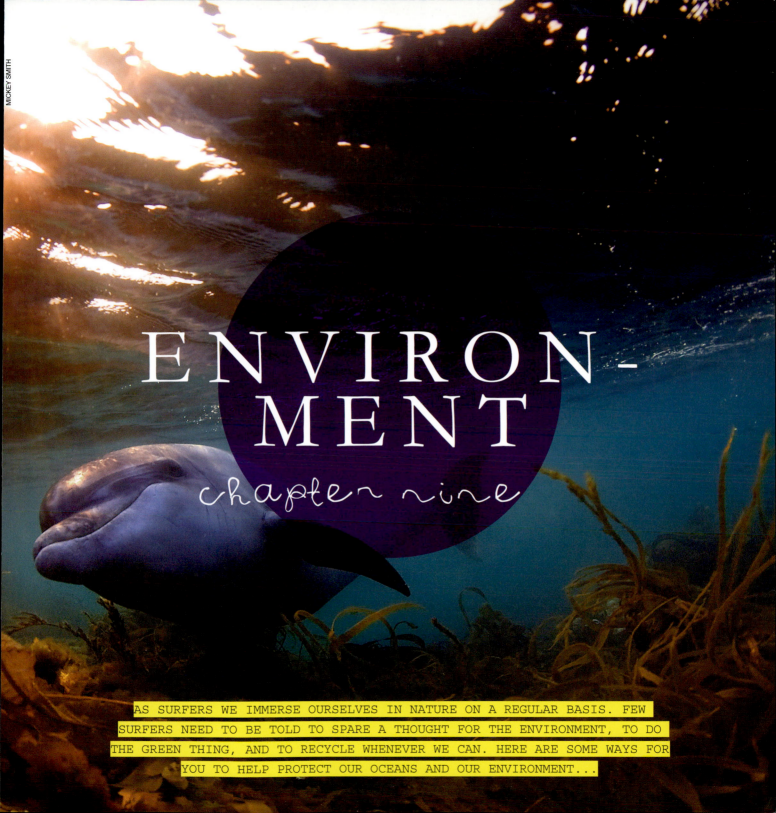

ENVIRON-MENT

chapter nine

AS SURFERS WE IMMERSE OURSELVES IN NATURE ON A REGULAR BASIS. FEW SURFERS NEED TO BE TOLD TO SPARE A THOUGHT FOR THE ENVIRONMENT, TO DO THE GREEN THING, AND TO RECYCLE WHENEVER WE CAN. HERE ARE SOME WAYS FOR YOU TO HELP PROTECT OUR OCEANS AND OUR ENVIRONMENT...

HEALTH OF THE OCEANS

Water covers nearly three-quarters of the Earth's surface, and a human body needs around two litres of the stuff per day. More than 97% of our entire planet's water is found in the ocean, which in turn provides 99% of the world's living space – making it the largest area in our universe inhabited by living creatures. But, although the oceans may be enormous, their health hangs in the balance.

REEF DESTRUCTION

Both rocky reefs and tropical coral reefs are fragile ecosystems that sustain life on planet Earth. Yes, they help create waves that you like to slide upon, but their contributions are far more important than providing our recreational environment.

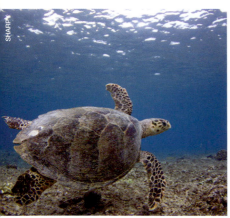

• Reefs protect shores from erosion by providing a barrier against the impact of waves and storms, while coral reefs – a living, breathing organism boasting some of the richest in biodiversity on the planet – offer benefits to humans in the form of food and medicine, and to sea creatures in the form of a nurturing habitat.

• Scientists estimate that more than 90% of marine species are directly or indirectly dependent on coral reefs. Among coral's biggest threats are pollution, overfishing, tourism, coastal development and bleaching (which occurs when corals are stressed by environmental conditions like unusually high sea temps, low salinity, and exposure to toxins). A recent World Wildlife Fund report estimated that 20% of the world's coral reefs have effectively been destroyed and show no immediate prospects of recovery, while half the world's coral reefs are under threat of collapse.

DO YOUR PART:

Reef Check (www.reefcheck.org) is a charity which organises teams of experienced recreational divers and village fishermen (who are trained and led by scientists) to produce relevant data, monitor reefs and facilitate conservation.

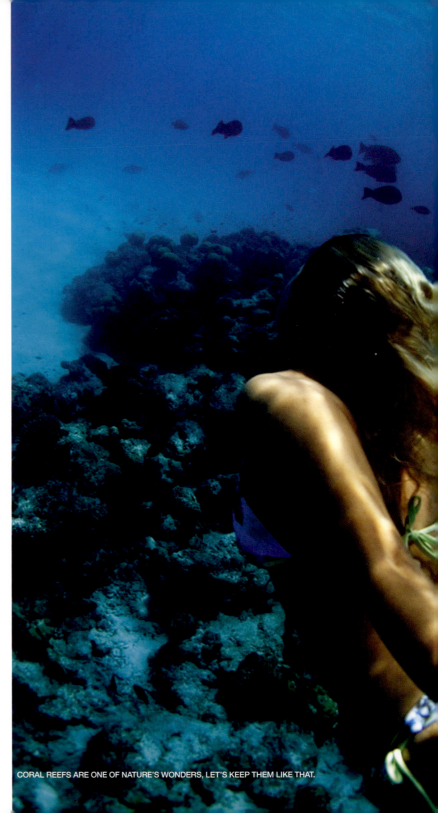

CORAL REEFS ARE ONE OF NATURE'S WONDERS, LET'S KEEP THEM LIKE THAT.

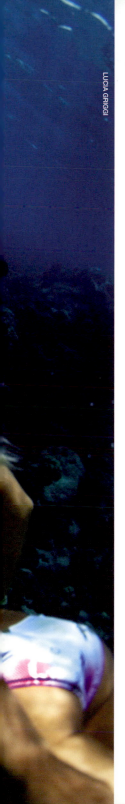

LUCIA GRIGGI

DECLINING FISH STOCKS

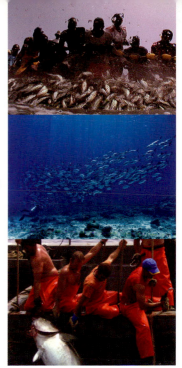

THE HARSH REALITY:

Our finned friends supply the greatest percentage of protein consumed by humans, yet most of the world's major fisheries are being fished beyond their sustainable yields. Due to our damaging practices, we're catching and killing fish faster than Mother Nature can replace them.

• The organisations Save the Sea (www.savethesea.org) estimates that more than 3.5 billion people depend on the ocean as their primary source of food, and that in 20 years this number could double to 7 billion. Populations of commercial favourites like tuna, cod, swordfish and marlin have declined by as much as 90% in the past century.

• Meanwhile, "by-catch" – the unintentional killing of species caused by the use of non-selective fishing gear like trawl nets, longlines and gillnets – amounts to 20 million tons of unnecessarily killed fish each year. The annual worldwide by-catch mortality of small whales, dolphins and porpoises alone is estimated to be more than 300,000.

DO YOUR PART:

Eat only sustainable seafood and refuse to eat actively endangered species, such as bluefin and bigeye tuna and skate. Put pressure on politicians to limit overfishing. Join the campaign to establish more marine reserves, where industrial fishing isn't allowed so fish stocks can replenish themselves.

WATER POLLUTION

COURTESY SAS

THE HARSH REALITY:

"When you think that our planet is covered in 72% water, one would think that rather than calling it Planet Earth we would call it Planet Ocean," says environmentalist David de Rothschild, whose Plastiki – a 60ft catamaran engineered from 12,500 reclaimed plastic bottles – journeyed more than 11,000 nautical miles from California to New South Wales to draw attention to the colossal amounts of plastic debris in our oceans.

• Scientists say that almost all of the marine pollution in the world is comprised of plastic materials, some of it smaller than the eye can see. Every year at least 1 million seabirds and 100,000 marine mammals and sea turtles die when they get caught in or ingest plastic waste.

• For surfers and sea creatures alike, chemical pollutants such as sewage and toxic chemicals are devastating too. While nasties might cause itchy eyes and dodgy tummies for wave riders, full-time water dwellers are being affected by harmful substances that tamper with their hormones. These so-called gender benders cause the feminisation of male fish and can be traced to everyday household cleaning products, shampoos, skin creams, washing detergents and paints.

DO YOUR PART:

Join and take part in the activities of the Surfrider Foundation (www.surfrider.org) and Surfers Against Sewage (www.sas.org.uk). "Not only are we here to help protect the health of surfers by campaigning for waters free from sewage effluent," says SAS Campaigns Officer Ruth Carruthers, "but we also help protect the environment and wildlife in a variety of other ways too, by working on issues such as climate change, safer shipping, hazardous chemicals, and carrying out regular beach cleans – making the beach a better place for everyone!"

HOW GREEN IS YOUR WAVE?

You may have noticed swell fanatics seem more concerned about the environment than non-surfers. Why? "Because we are immersed in nature," says Animal team rider Easkey Britton, who holds four Irish National Championships and an honours degree in environmental science. "It's the heightened awareness of the ocean's moods and seasons and how that effects us that makes us take more notice," she continues. "We're also much more exposed to the damage we cause as humans. I've got sick from pollution and untreated waste at some of my favourite surf breaks. We see dolphins and sea life washed ashore tangled in gill nets or suffocated from plastic bags. So the harmful impacts on the environment aren't abstract to us, they're real because we experience them first hand."

The irony is though that pursuing a passion for waves has a carbon footprint implication. What's a girl to do? You can start by following these tips for countering climate change as you search out swells…

BRUCE BROWN HAS A LOT TO ANSWER FOR. His

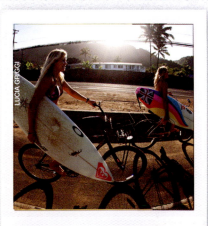

1964 classic, *The Endless Summer*, practically invented the concept of surf travel, and board riders ever since have yearned to join the surfing jet set. If you're lucky enough to fly to far-flung waters this year, reduce the damage of your air travel by buying carbon offsets when you book: www.carbonfootprint.com.

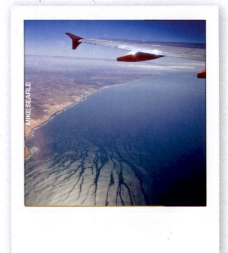

MIKE SEARLE

WAX ON, WAX OFF – OR SO A WISE MAN ONCE SAID. The truth is that wax has a way of working itself off your board and into the water, where it can harm those who make the ocean their home. Opt for biodegradable, petroleum-free and non-toxic versions like Treehugger Surf Wax or Matunas biodegradable surf wax.

AS QUIVER CARRIERS GO, A VEHICLE WITH FOUR WHEELS IS HARD TO BEAT, AND SOMETIMES THERE'S NO BETTER WAY TO SCOUT THE BEST BREAK ON THE DAY THAN BY CAR. So if you must drive be efficient about it. Consult maps and guidebooks beforehand to minimise wrong turns. The latest Wavefinder guide is great, and how's this for a tree-friendly feature: you can buy chapters online as PDFs then print only the pages you need at www.wave-finder.com.

If you want to rip harder, then drive less – and run, skate and cycle more. Give Lush's Samba skate a whirl; it's the ideal choice for a longboard that behaves like a surfboard. www.lushlongboards.com.

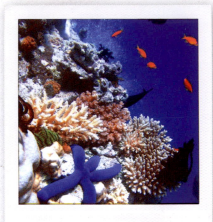

CORAL IS A HANDY LITTLE ORGANISM, PRODUCING PEELING RIGHTS AND SPITTING TUBES FROM COSTA RICA TO BALI. But scientists say there's a link between dying coral reefs and the 6,000 tons of sunscreen that slides off our skin annually. Play it safe and use plant and mineral-based rather petroleum-derived products, and rely on physical barriers that reflect UV rays instead of chemical ones that work by absorbing radiation. Active ingredients zinc oxide or titanium dioxide are the ones you want – try Trevarno's SPF15 Elements Balm - it combats wetsuit chafing too (www.trevarnoskincare.co.uk) or Mexitan's reef friendly products (www.mexitan.com).

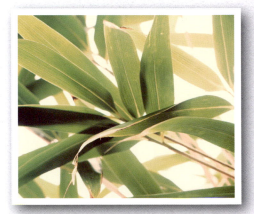

TO DRESS FOR THE PLANET'S SUCCESS, GO GREEN IN THE WATER. Xcel's latest Infiniti and Drylock suits feature earth-friendly lining made from bamboo charcoal that's been fused with recycled fibres. While Rip Curl Planet swimsuits are made from recycled polyester.

LUCIA GRIGGI

If you're literally sick and tired of dodging chemical pollutants and plastic, then join the efforts of Surfers Against Sewage (www.sas.org.uk) or Surfrider Foundation (www.surfrider.com). "The effort to secure healthy coastal water quality comes down to one thing: the individual," says Surfrider Foundation's Matt McClain. "The choices we make as individuals are what make the biggest impact on coastal water quality." Take action through membership, events, fundraising and campaigns.

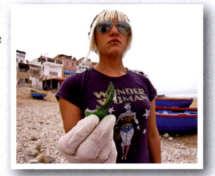

GOOD GEAR DOES NOT BELONG IN THE LANDFILL. Modern surfboards and wetsuits are built to last, not break down, so if you've got old kit, sell it or give it away. Post your pre-loved booty on Secondhandboards.com or Rerip.com, and donate old wetsuits to Rip Curl's Project Resurrection, which sees old neoprene reborn as sandals.

FOR LAND-LOCKED SURFERS PLANNING A DOMESTIC GETAWAY, INCORPORATE A RIDE-SHARING SCHEME INTO YOUR EXIT STRATEGY. Groups like the London Surf Club offer online forums to coordinate drivers and riders, while the Big Friday bus ferries London surfers to breaks on a weekly basis in the summer. Find out more at www.bigfriday.com.

The pure pursuit of surfing has a seriously ugly underside. Until recently pretty much all boards contained polyester resin, toluene, polyurethane and polystyrene – a cocktail of toxic non-biodegradable fossil-fuel nasties that release huge amounts of CO_2 during production. But there is hope on the horizon in the form of plant-derived foam blanks, epoxy and linseed oil resins, recyclable EPS foam cores and bamboo. Check out these boards – Country Feeling Surfboards in Hawaii, Tiki in the UK and Firewire which are available globally, and if you add OAM's new 100% recycled traction pad and Green Flex fins by FCS, then you'll be throwing your spray using reclaimed bits of shoes, sandals and carpet fibres too.

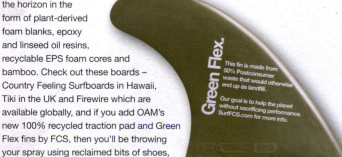

OCEAN CRUSADERS

Help out by helping the organisations who strive to protect our oceans. Here's a few of the organisations working hard on your behalf...

THE SURFRIDER FOUNDATION is a non-profit grassroots organization dedicated to the protection and enjoyment of our world's oceans, waves and beaches. Founded in 1984 by a handful of visionary surfers in Malibu, California, the Surfrider Foundation now has over 50,000 members and 90 chapters worldwide. www.surfrider.com

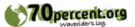

70PERCENT: 70percent was built to help small groups of friends share knowledge built from years of studying and riding waves and to promote water quality awareness. www.70percent.org/blog

SAVE THE WAVES COALITION is an environmental coalition dedicated to preserving the world's surf spots and their surrounding environments. Their goal is to protect surfing locations around the planet and to educate the public about their value. Save the Waves works in partnership with local communities, foreign and national governments, as well as other conservation groups to prevent coastal developments from damaging the surf zone. www.savethewaves.org

SURFERS AGAINST SEWAGE campaign for clean and safe recreational water, free from sewage effluents, toxic chemicals, nuclear waste and marine litter in the UK. www.sas.org.uk

SURFERS FOR CETACEANS call on surfers everywhere to support the conservation and protection of whales and dolphins and other marine wildlife, to protest whaling and the killing of threatened and endangered species, and to end the pollution of our marine environment. www.surfersforcetaceans.com

SEA SHEPHERD CONSERVATION SOCIETY. Established in 1977, the Sea Shepherd Conservation Society (SSCS) is an international non-profit, marine wildlife conservation organisation. Their mission is to end the destruction of habitat and slaughter of wildlife in the world's oceans and to conserve and protect ecosystems and species. www.seashepherd.com

SURFERS ENVIRONMENTAL ALLIANCE (SEA) was founded by surfers who wanted to do something to protect the ocean, beaches and coastlines, and keep this planet a safe place to surf. If you own a surfboard, enjoy the beauty of the ocean, or if you are concerned about preserving our ocean planet, get involved with SEA. www.seasurfer.org

UPCYCLING

Get in on the upcycling act and help keep rubbish out of our ocean and landfills. Here's how to turn trash into treasure.

We all want to be 'greener' but is 'just' recycling enough these days? It requires energy to ship those bottles, newspapers and cans abroad, to break them down and to build them back up into something new again. And there are still plenty of substances around that can't easily be recycled — neoprene for example.

If you're looking to 'do your bit' a bit more, then get your head around upcycling. Upcycling basically means taking something and finding a new use for it when it's served its original purpose — thus extending the lifespan of existing resources without further taxing the planet.

CREATIVE THINKING

Upcycling isn't complicated. When a beachside cafe covers an old surfboard in blackboard paint and reinvents it as their Special's Board: that's upcycling. It inherently involves a creative challenge, because to reinvent an object as a new 'useful' thing requires imagination. Who would have thought that juice bottle would look good as a plant pot?!

Fortunately creativity is something that surfers seem to have in a healthy supply. Riding a wave requires a surfer to look at what's available and decide in a split-second how to make the most of it — maybe this explains why surfing attracts a disproportionate number of creative people, such as artists, musicians and photographers...

And maybe it explains why there are so many examples of upcycling in the surf world. In Cuba, for example — where resources are incredibly limited due to the US trade embargo — shapers rescue foam from the inside of refrigerators to use as blanks for

surfboards: definitely a 'cool' board! At the other end of a board's life you'll find Welsh product designer Adam Scott, who upcycles old sticks into seating. (www.surfchair.co.uk)

The clever people at Green Guru Gear have experimented with reclaiming billboards to create durable board bags, while Looptworks turn neoprene salvaged from wetsuit manufacturers into shockproof laptop sleeves. (www.greengurugear.com; www.looptworks.com)

FASHION FRIENDLY

Upcycling has many uses, ranging from the practical to the fashionable. Odd Socks are a Cornish company who make board socks from unloved and redundant 1970s curtains that they hunt down at boot sales and charity shops – the crazier the better! (www.oddsocks.moonfruit.com). And at the cutting-edge of the "trashion" movement is Beck(y), an outfit that upcylces old skate decks into accessories (www.beckycity.com).

Of course, reuse is such a good idea that it's not just the little guys who are doing it. Major players in the surf world are busy recycling PET plastic into boardies and bikinis, while Resurf has figured out a way to break down old boards so that they can be reborn as an element of the concrete and asphalt mixes that make up our road surfaces.

If you need some upcycling inspiration for your own small-scale projects, then visit www.Korduroy.tv for a host of surf-centric projects. Their Surf Sufficient channel features videos that show you how to use bits of old surf wax to make beer mats, how to employ not-too-tatty old tights in the noble pursuit of wax removal, and how a couple of five litre water bottles can help keep you toastie after that February dawnie...

THE CHANGE GAME

If you have scissors and a sewing machine and can lay down straight lines of stitching, then here are three upcycling projects to keep you busy.

A **Sew two old towels together along their longest sides, then add a drawstring at the top to create a mobile changing robe.** By poking your head out the top and tightening the drawstring, you can strip out of bikini bottoms with your modesty still intact.

B **An underutilised yoga mat can be called in to car park detail too.** Cut it to fit the seat of your car to protect the dry interior from your damp posterior. Another piece on the ground will keep the chill of morning concrete from your toes, and prevent sand and soil from sticking to your salty extremities.

C **Cut the arms off an old fleece jacket and sew the sleeves shut at the cut end.** Stick an empty water bottle – preferably the 1 litre sport size with squirt top – into each 'sleeve tube', then tie a cord around the neck. Half fill the bottles with hot tap water, then top up with boiled water. Use your new hot water bottles to warm your wettie, then utilise the squirt function at the end of your sessions for an impromptu shower.

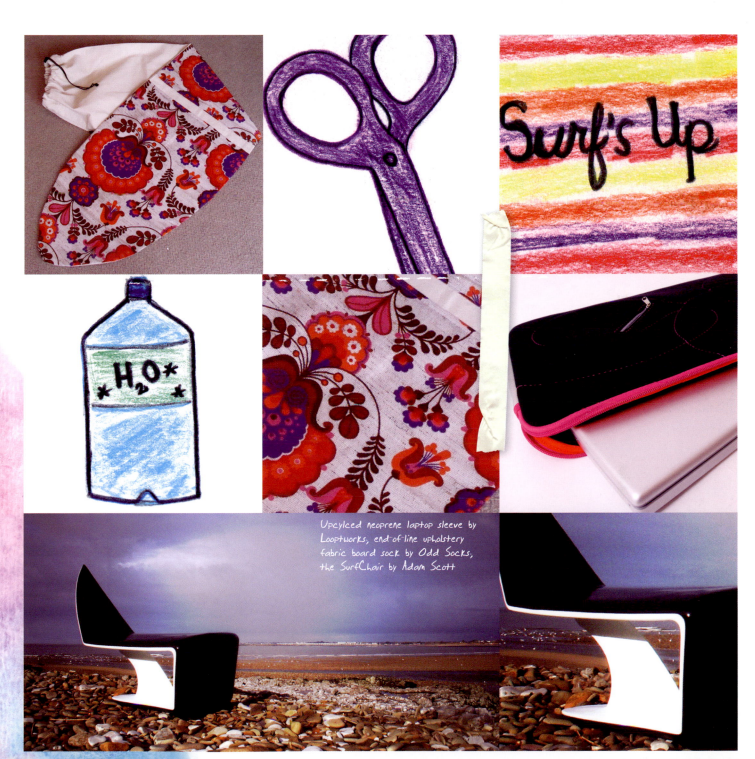

Upcylced neoprene laptop sleeve by Looptworks; end-of-line upholstery fabric board sock by Odd Socks; the SurfChair by Adam Scott

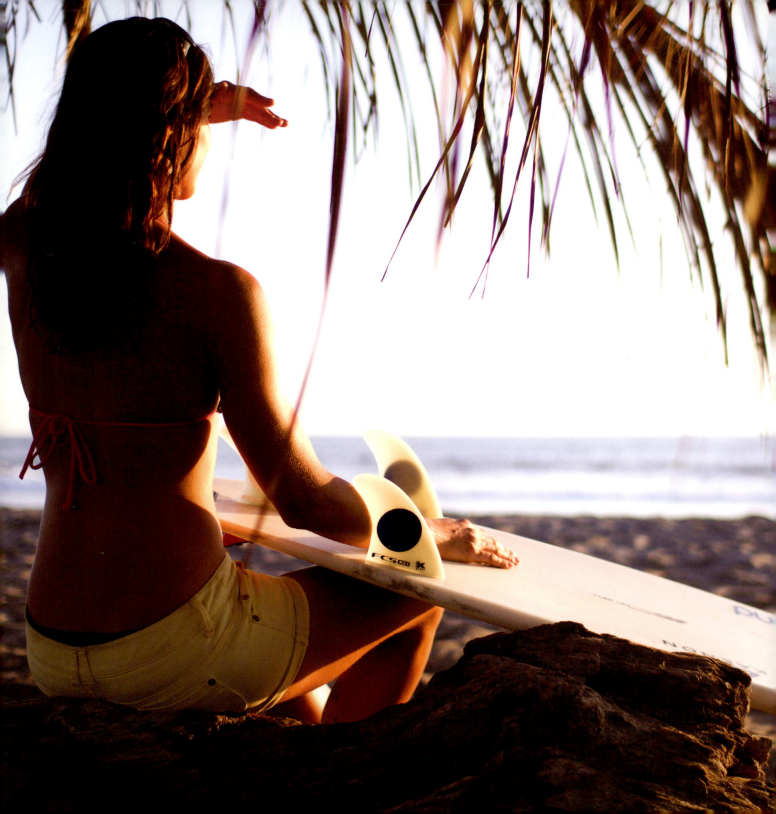

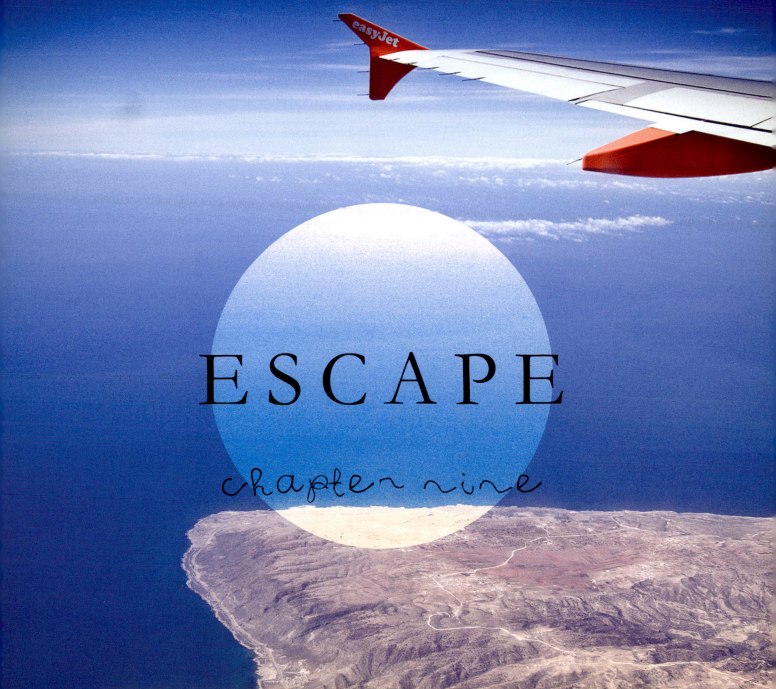

ESCAPE

chapter nine

TO TRAVEL IS TO ENRICH YOUR EXISTENCE, TO OPEN YOUR MIND TO WAYS OF LIFE FAR REMOVED FROM YOUR OWN. AMIDST EVERYTHING YOU EXPERIENCE WHEN YOU TRAVEL – THE ONE THING THAT REALLY GETS THE HEART POUNDING IS FINDING PERFECT WAVES ON FAR FLUNG SHORES...

12 CLASSIC DESTINATIONS

'So many waves, so little time', is the oft-quoted mantra of the surf traveller. Luckily cheap flights and tailor-made holidays mean that 24 hours after reading this you could be on the other side of the globe having the best surf of your life!

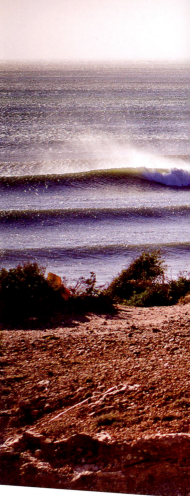

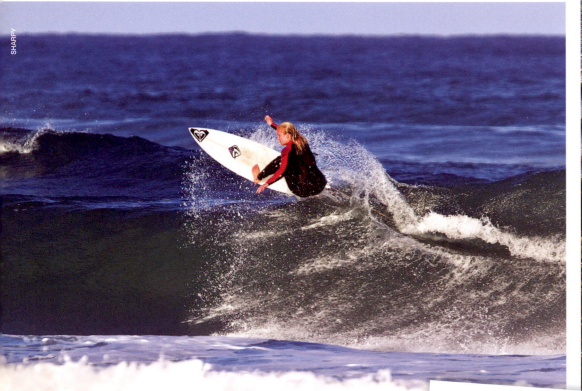

GABI ROWE IN SOUTH WEST PORTUGAL.

■ PORTUGAL

■ **What to expect** Surprisingly cool water, punchy beachbreaks and some lovely long wrapping points. Portugal's long coast has something for everyone.

■ **When to go** The best time of year is March to September.

■ **Where to surf** The warm Algarve coast has a great variety of beaches for beginners and some nice waves for advanced surfers. The more rugged reefs of Ericeira produce some challenging conditions for advanced surfers. Peniche has some great waves for beginners, and Supertubos for the advanced surfer. Peniche also has the added advantage of being located on a peninsula so no matter what the wind direction there is usually somewhere to surf.

■ **What will £20 buy you?** The Portuguese love to party and the coolest Portuguese clubs don't get started until at least 1am. £20 would pay for (some of!) a night on the tiles. If it's flat check out Lisbon, it's one of the grandest cities in Europe (just avoid the roads during rush hour).

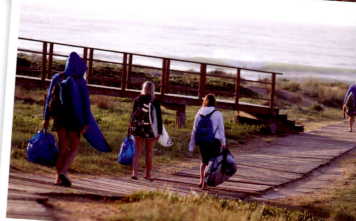

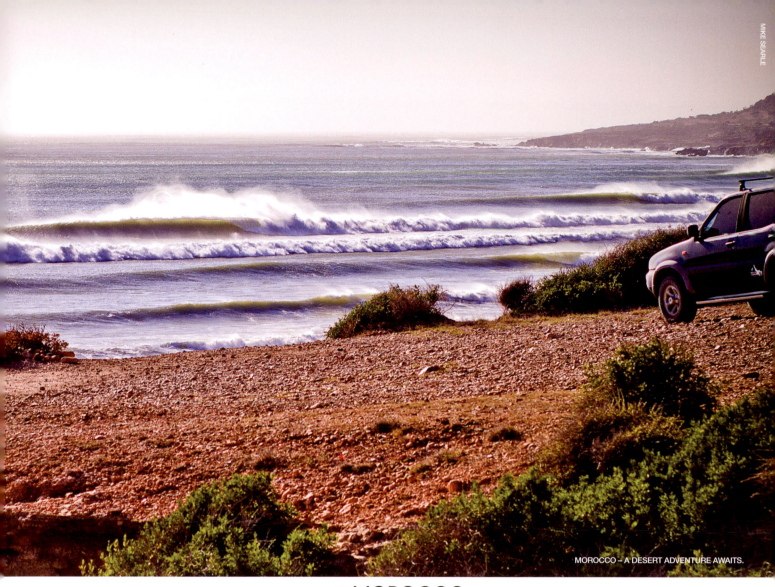

MIKE SEARLE

MOROCCO – A DESERT ADVENTURE AWAITS.

■ MOROCCO

■ **What to expect** Deep in the heart of North Africa there is a fishing village called Taghazout, just north of Agadir, which comes alive each winter with the sound of pounding pointbreaks and surf banter. It's a beautiful place with a rich Arabic culture to add to the magic.

■ **When to go** October to April. With December, January and February being the pick of the months.

■ **Where to surf** There are several beachbreaks south of Taghazout suitable for beginners. Intermediates and experts can take advantage of pointbreaks like Killers and Anchor Point which are suitable for intermediate surfers when small, but can also hold waves big enough to test any expert.

■ **What will £20 buy you?** At one of the Souks (local markets) you could get all manner of local trinkets, knitted bags and funky presents for everyone at home.

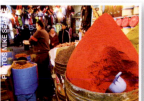
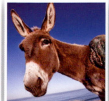
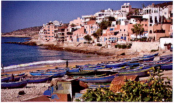

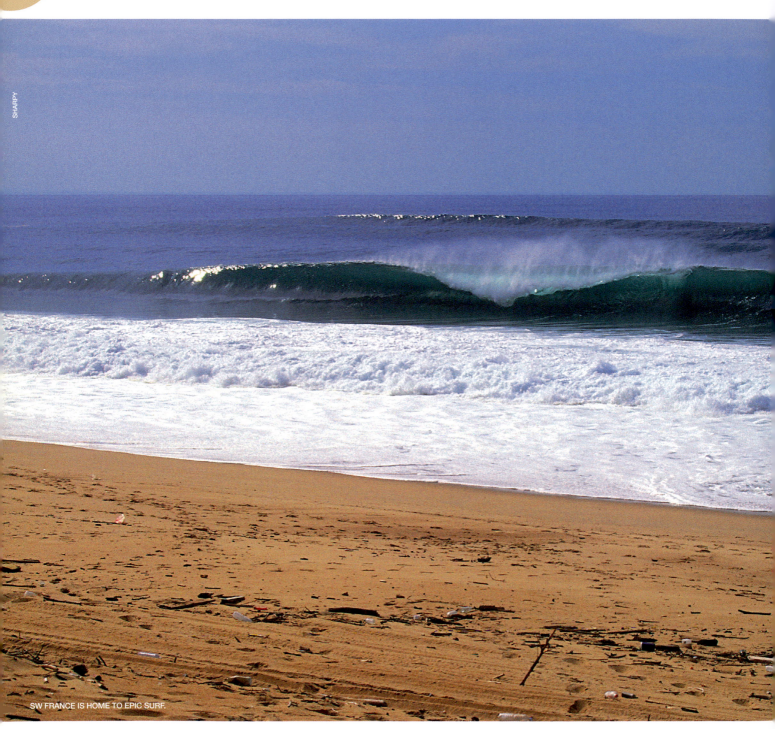

SHARPY

SW FRANCE IS HOME TO EPIC SURF.

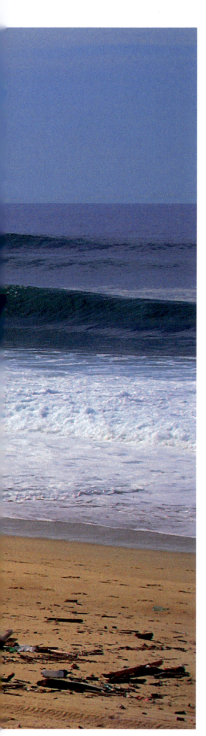

FRANCE

■ **What to expect** Head for Hossegor and you'll find ten kilometres of the best beachbreaks in the world. Graviere, La Nord, Estagnots and Bourdaines are names that roll off the tongue and stir the blood of surfers across Europe. Expect perfect beachbreak peaks and a hardcore party atmosphere throughout the autumn and winter seasons.

■ **When to go** The deep water trench located off the Landes coast sucks every morsel of swell from the Atlantic Ocean and focuses it on the hard shallow sands. Autumn is best for swell so try to hit the area in September when the summer's warmth is still in the air and water, yet the crowds are heading home.

■ **Where to surf** Finding the waves is easy, just pick your favourite spot and check it. If it's no good, just choose a direction, north or south, and walk.

It the weather and swell patterns are in place, you won't be disappointed. Les Estagnots is a favourite, as is Le Penon.

■ **What will £20 buy you?** If you do fail in your mission to find waves, head for the roadside coffee bars and then venture forth to legendary nightspots like Rock Food or Dick's Sand Bar. Just don't plan much surfing the next day! For £20 you'll get a nice meal and a couple of beers at Le Surfing in Les Estagnots.

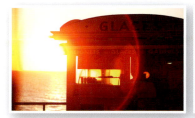
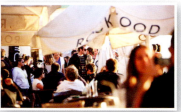
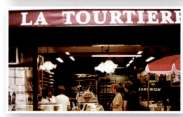
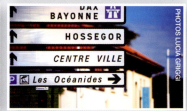

PHOTOS LUCIA GRIGGI

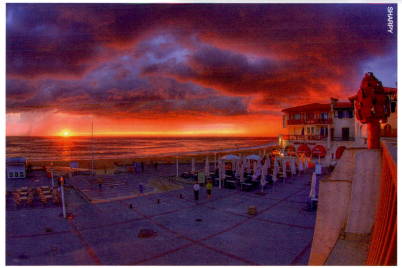

SHARPY

GREAT SURF, GOOD FOOD AND AN AWESOME PARTY DESTINATION, SW FRANCE HAS A LOT GOING FOR IT.

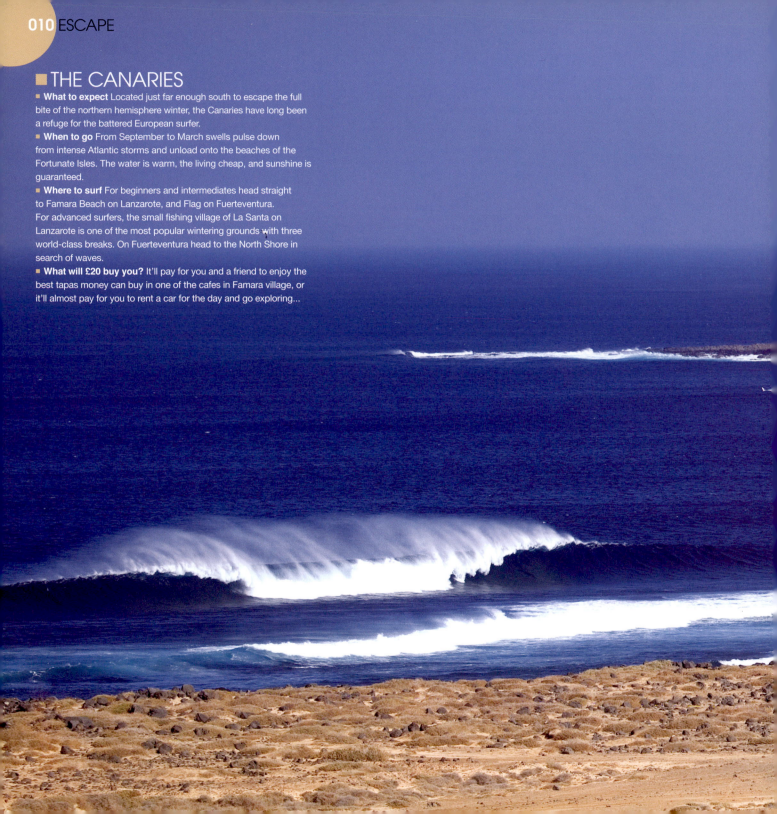

THE CANARIES

- **What to expect** Located just far enough south to escape the full bite of the northern hemisphere winter, the Canaries have long been a refuge for the battered European surfer.
- **When to go** From September to March swells pulse down from intense Atlantic storms and unload onto the beaches of the Fortunate Isles. The water is warm, the living cheap, and sunshine is guaranteed.
- **Where to surf** For beginners and intermediates head straight to Famara Beach on Lanzarote, and Flag on Fuerteventura. For advanced surfers, the small fishing village of La Santa on Lanzarote is one of the most popular wintering grounds with three world-class breaks. On Fuerteventura head to the North Shore in search of waves.
- **What will £20 buy you?** It'll pay for you and a friend to enjoy the best tapas money can buy in one of the cafes in Famara village, or it'll almost pay for you to rent a car for the day and go exploring...

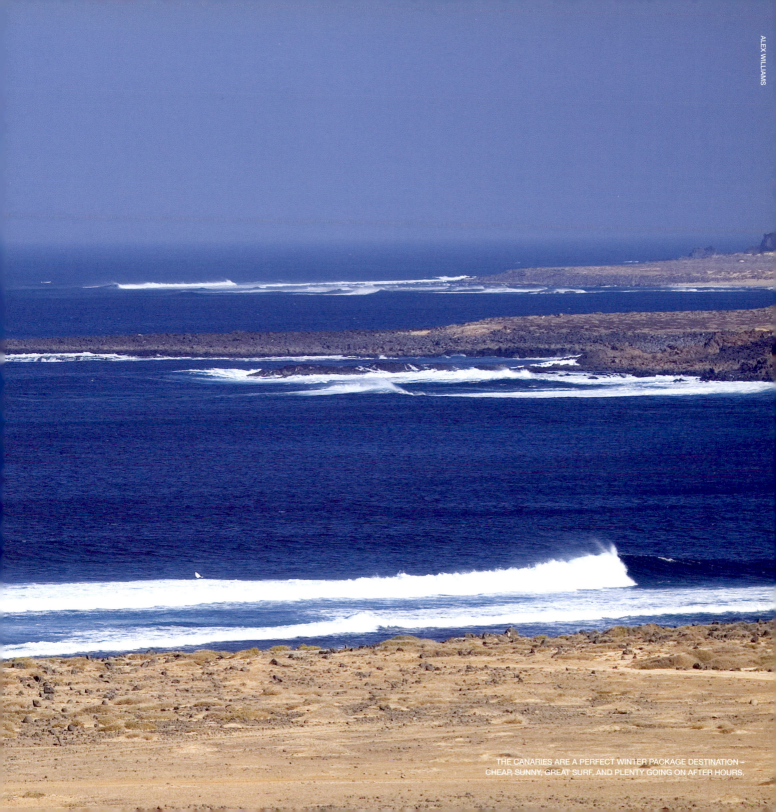

THE CANARIES ARE A PERFECT WINTER PACKAGE DESTINATION –
CHEAP, SUNNY, GREAT SURF, AND PLENTY GOING ON AFTER HOURS.

CALIFORNIA

■ **What to expect** California boasts some prime surfing spots, more McDonalds than you could visit in a lifetime, and more beautiful people than you could ever imagine.

■ **When to go** In the winter you'll need a 3mm full suit. In the summer you just need a short sleeve spring suit. The non-wuss can go without a suit during July and August. Winter's probably the best for surf – La Jolla really ropes in the swell plus there's snow in the mountains. The weather is super nice with lots of sun and temperature getting up to around 20°C.

■ **Where to surf** Beginner and intermediate surfers could battle the crowds at beachbreaks such as Huntington Beach. Advanced surfers should head for the numerous reefbreaks of La Jolla and one of the best beachbreaks – Black's.

■ **What will £20 buy you?** About ten gut-plugging Burritos, eight McDonald's cheeseburgers, two CDs, enough petrol to drive to the mountains and back in the winter to go snowboarding, or petrol and insurance for a day trip into Mexico for a surf.

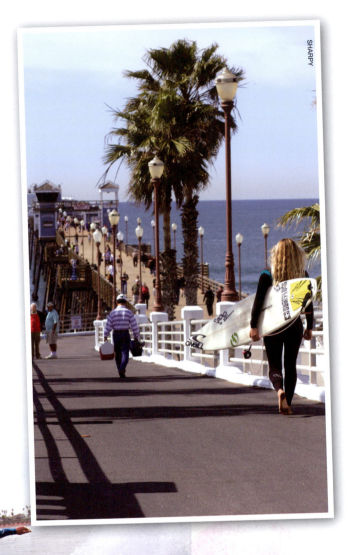

CALIFORNIA OFFERS A PERFECT BALANCE OF SURFING AND FUN.

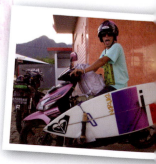

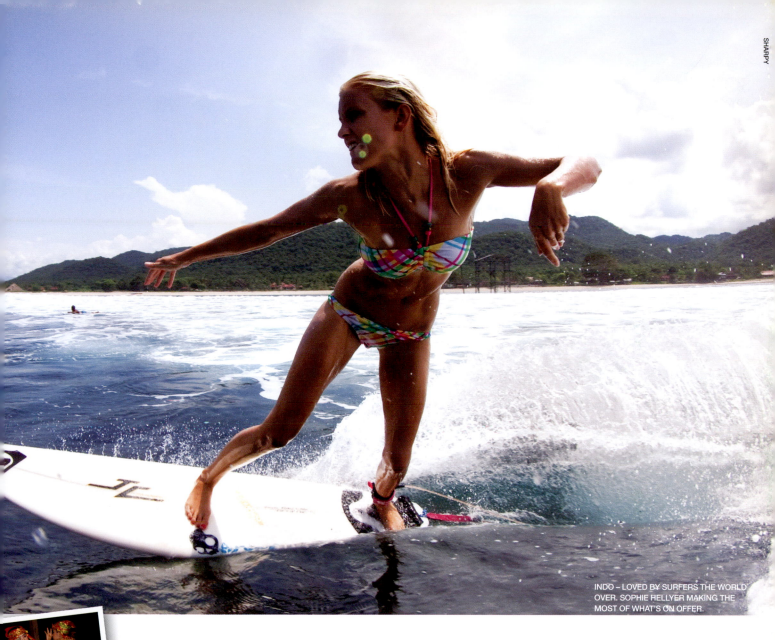

INDO – LOVED BY SURFERS THE WORLD OVER. SOPHIE HELLYER MAKING THE MOST OF WHAT'S ON OFFER.

■ BALI, INDONESIA

■ **What to expect** There are many perfect waves within the archipelago of Indonesia that could make this list but Bali is still the Island of the Gods. Despite the horrific bombing of Kuta in 2003, the island is still a very special place. The hospitality of the people, beauty of the countryside and perfect waves make it a magical place. And, although most of the famous waves break over sharp shallow coral reefs, there are also a number of beachbreaks suitable for beginners and intermediates.

■ **When to go** May to November is the dry season when the waves seem to be offshore every day and it never rains. You can score waves year round though.

■ **Where to surf Beginners** – Kuta and Legian Beaches offer great waves for learning, but watch out for rips. Intermediates – Dreamland and Cangu offer more of a challenge with the long rivermouth waves of Medawai offering an adventure. **Advanced** – Uluwatu, Padang Padang, Bingin, Nusa Dua, Sanur - take your pick!

■ **What will £20 buy you?** Twenty sarongs, four slap-up meals or you could get your hair platted and your nails painted every day for a week!

SOUTH AFRICA

■ **What to expect** Africa – just the word conjures up images of adventure. To the surfer, Africa means Durban, Cape Town and one wave in particular: the princess of the south, Jeffrey's Bay. A small town now surrounds the legendary wave that has become a Mecca for surfers around the globe.

■ **When to go** Best season: April- July, but there are waves all year round in Cape Town and Durban.

■ **Where to surf** Beginners should check out North Beach in Durban for plenty of fun peaks. Intermediates can head for the shelving waves of Ballito and the Umhlanga Rocks area. Advanced surfers should check out J-Bay. At its best J-Bay is all things to all surfers, a long wave with plenty of room for manoeuvres, tube riding and speed. Cold and often windy (from the storms needed to produce the optimum surf conditions) this is not the place to go to bask on the beach.

■ **What will £20 buy you?** The close proximity of the world renowned national wildlife parks, mean lounging around and sunbathing should be low on your list of priorities. £20 will pay for an unforgettable wildlife-checking day out.

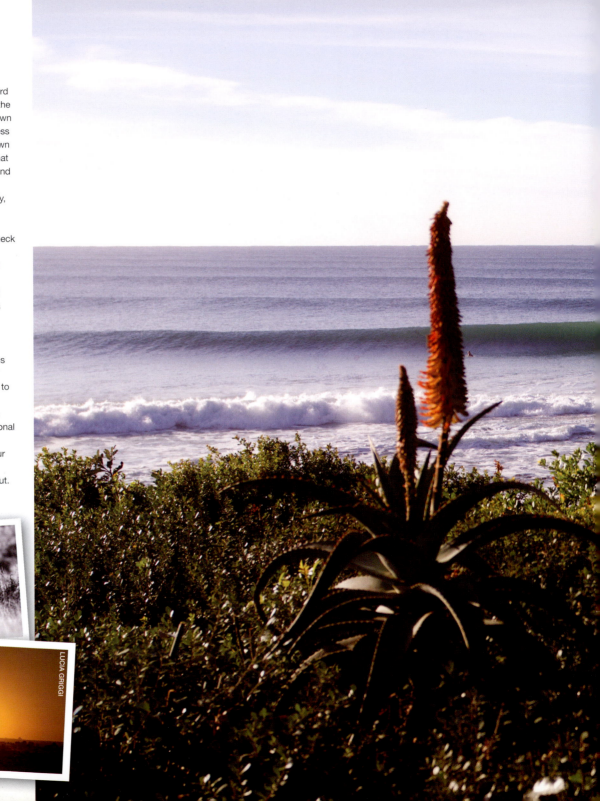

LUCIA GRIGGI

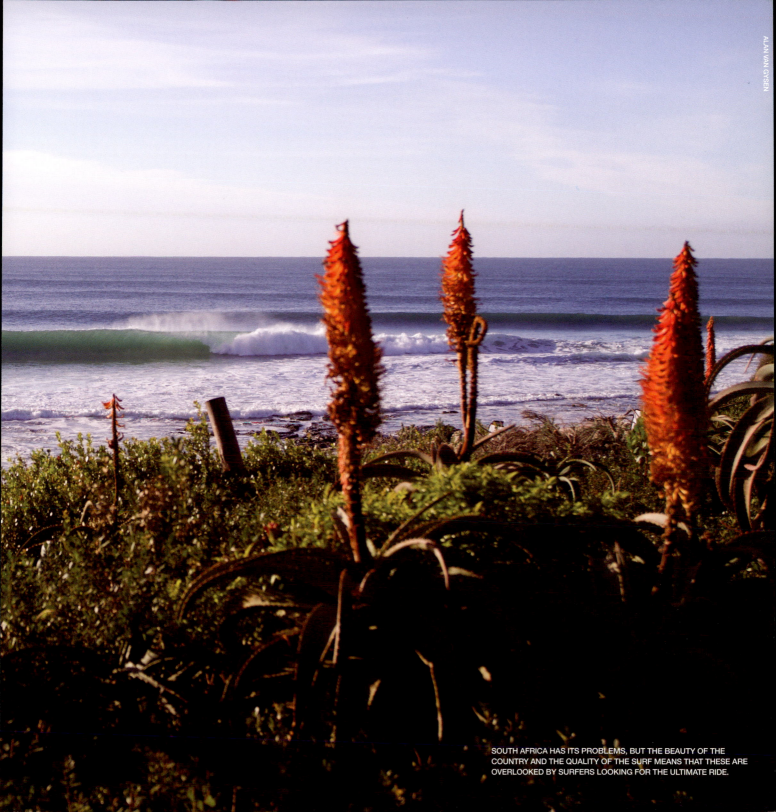

SOUTH AFRICA HAS ITS PROBLEMS, BUT THE BEAUTY OF THE
COUNTRY AND THE QUALITY OF THE SURF MEANS THAT THESE ARE
OVERLOOKED BY SURFERS LOOKING FOR THE ULTIMATE RIDE.

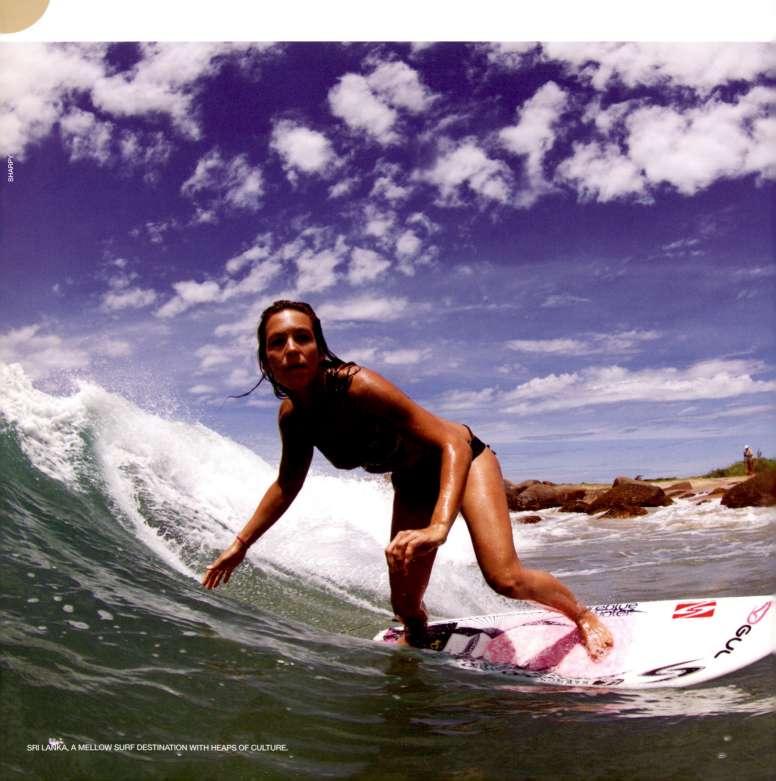

SHARPY

SRI LANKA, A MELLOW SURF DESTINATION WITH HEAPS OF CULTURE.

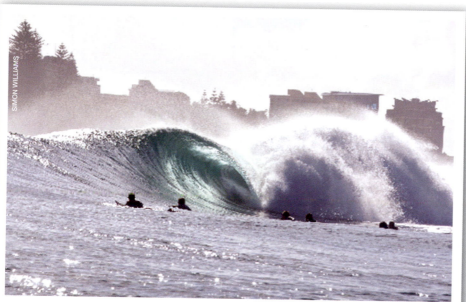

AUSTRALIA

- **What to expect** The pointbreaks of Kirra, Burleigh Heads and Greenmount on Australia's Gold Coast are some of the surfing world's great natural wonders. If you want to enjoy them at their best though you'll have to set your alarm clock, as the coast has now taken over from Malibu as one of the most crowded surf areas on earth. However there are so many beaches you'll still find plenty of room. And if it goes flat, well, this is Australia's favourite holiday destination so there's plenty more to do.
- **When to go** January to April is generally the best time to visit the Gold Coast.
- **Where to surf** Beginners and intermediates just pick a beach. There are miles and miles of beaches suitable for learning. For advanced surfers, The Superbank – stretching from Snapper Rocks, through Rainbow Bay to Kirra – is world famous but very crowded. Burleigh Heads and Currumbin offer great alternatives.
- **What will £20 buy you?** From sports fishing to the multiplex cinemas, bars, nightclubs, golf courses and the most varied selection of restaurants, there's plenty to spend your money on. £20 will get you entry into the cinema followed by a light snack at Sushi Train afterwards.

SRI LANKA

- **What to expect** A surfer's escape since the 70s, Sri Lanka has plenty of waves, picture perfect beaches, a friendly vibe and plenty of culture.
- **When to go** There are two distinct seasons: December to March when the wind is offshore on the west coast breaks of Hikadua and Midigama, and the southwest monsoon (June to October) when Arugam Bay and the east coast goes off.
- **Where to surf** On the east side, centred around Hikkadua, beaches and reefs dominate. On the western side there is the occasional reef, but it's mainly long sand points, which are good for intermediates. Head to Arugam Bay as it's the best swell magnet of all the points and you can almost always guarantee that The Point will be a couple of feet bigger than any of the other breaks. But watch out for crowds. Also check out Pottuvil Point – it's every surfer's dream tropical wave.
- **What will £20 buy you?** Dinner at a beach side café and enough saris to keep you happy for years.

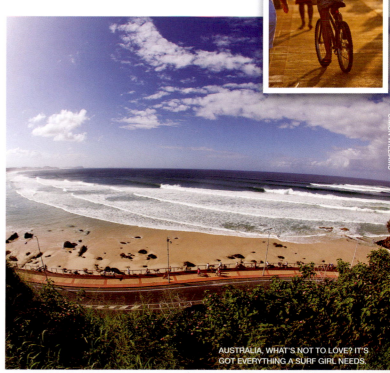

AUSTRALIA, WHAT'S NOT TO LOVE? IT'S GOT EVERYTHING A SURF GIRL NEEDS.

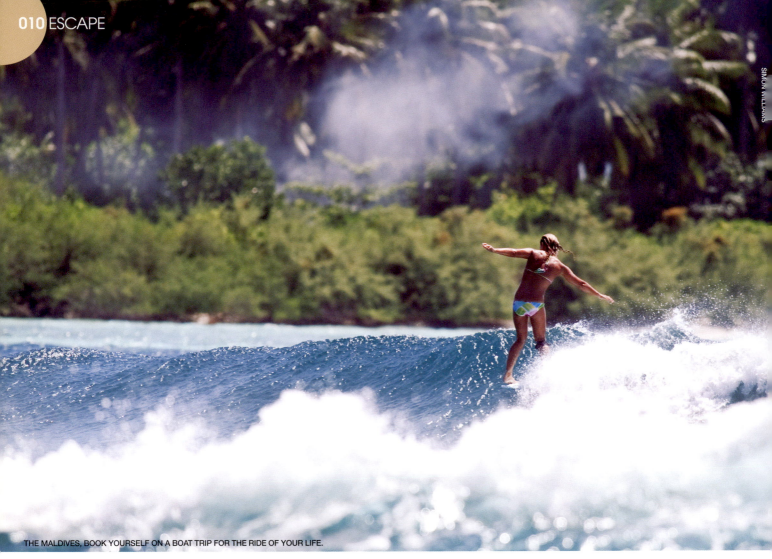

SIMON WILLIAMS

THE MALDIVES, BOOK YOURSELF ON A BOAT TRIP FOR THE RIDE OF YOUR LIFE.

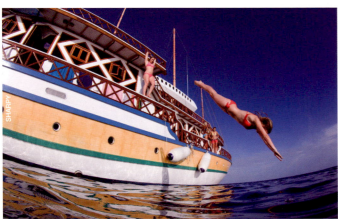

SHARPY

THE MALDIVES

For a luxury surf trip you'll never forget, the Maldives is all time. The Maldives are situated just north of the equator, off the southern tip of India. Depending on your definition of 'island', there are upwards of 1,000 islands in the archipelago, although most are tiny uninhabited coral atolls.

■ **When to go** The biggest and most consistent swell is between March and October but anytime is good and it's bikinis all year round but you might want to wear a shortie to protect your skin from the reef.

■ **Where to surf** For a hassle-free adventure choose a boat trip or a resort that will ferry you to the waves. The Maldives are separated into North and South Atolls with the south/southeast facing reefs on the southern atolls get the best surf.

■ **What will £20 buy you?** Not a lot as most stuff is imported so it's all expensive. The word budget and Maldives don't really go together well.

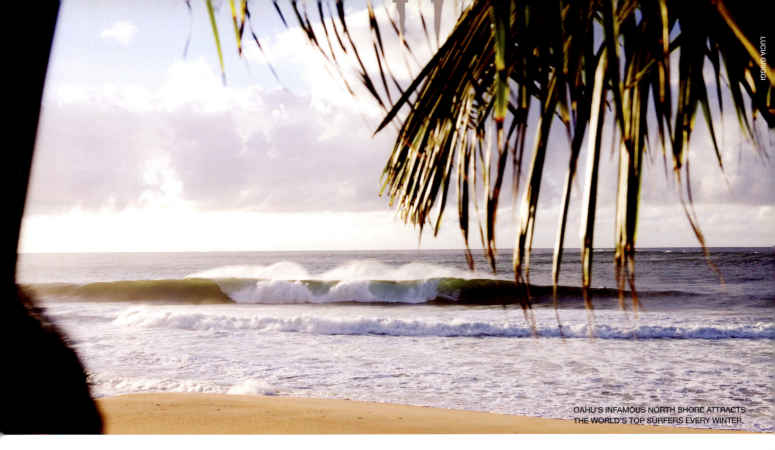

LUCIA GRIGGI

OAHU'S INFAMOUS NORTH SHORE ATTRACTS THE WORLD'S TOP SURFERS EVERY WINTER.

■ HAWAII

■ **What to expect** This ten-mile stretch of coast contains some of the best surf spots on earth. Pipeline, Sunset, and Waimea Bay are the places where legends have been created and reputations built. Huge swells derived from north Pacific storms radiate down and slam into the volcanic island chain, producing surf that is larger and more powerful than anywhere else on earth. It's where the final leg of the men's pro tour comes to town to crown its World Champion at the Banzai Pipeline, a gladiatorial pit that breaks just metres from the shore. And on the beach the atmosphere is almost as electric as in the ocean.

■ **When to go** From November to March.

■ **Where to surf** For beginners and intermediates it tends to be spectating only, apart from really small days when Ehukai Beach park is fun. Also check out Monster Mush or V-Land when the swell is small and manageable.

■ **What will £20 buy you?** It'll buy two of you breakfast in the Café Haleiwa and you'll hear all about that morning's exploits straight from the horse's mouths: the heroics, the performances and the horror stories!

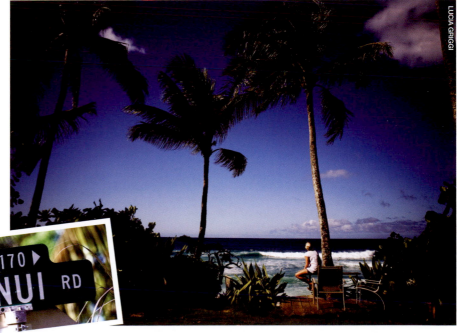

LUCIA GRIGGI

59-170 ▶
KE NUI RD

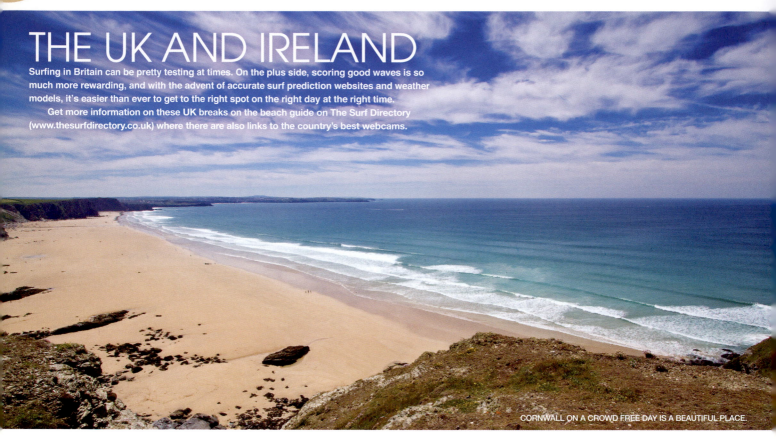

THE UK AND IRELAND

Surfing in Britain can be pretty testing at times. On the plus side, scoring good waves is so much more rewarding, and with the advent of accurate surf prediction websites and weather models, it's easier than ever to get to the right spot on the right day at the right time.

Get more information on these UK breaks on the beach guide on The Surf Directory (www.thesurfdirectory.co.uk) where there are also links to the country's best webcams.

CORNWALL ON A CROWD FREE DAY IS A BEAUTIFUL PLACE.

CORNWALL

Arguably Britain's best stretch of coastline, the Cornish coast probably receives the most consistent surf in the country. With a healthy population of local surf girls there'll be no shortage of inspiration either, and a great selection of open aspect beaches which pick up any swell from passing lows.

Fistral is one of Cornwall's most consistent surf spots, which works at all states of the tide and with plenty of channels to paddle out. Because of that the main hazard at this break is the crowds! Head out of Newquay in the summer to avoid the crowds and you'll find plenty of beachbreaks and reefs to suit most levels. Constantine offers less crowded surf and a varied array of good waves, or head further west to investigate some of the coves and bays further along the Cornish peninsula.

On the south coast Praa Sands works well on big southwest swells when the north shore is blown out. There's a fast sucky shorey towards neap high tide with manageable 'learner slopes' at other stages of the tide. Porthleven is the jewel in the south coast's crown – a top-quality reef that holds waves up to 12 feet. It works best when there's a deep low sitting around the Bay of Biscay, and a northeasterly wind. Best from mid to three quarters tide and definitely for experienced surfers only.

If you're a learner head to the gently-shelving beaches of Towan, Great Western and Tolcarne in Newquay Bay. They are sheltered from the brunt of Atlantic swells, so are ideal places to build your confidence and practice your moves!

DEVON

North Devon is a top quality surfing destination with Croyde at the epicentre. It can get pretty crowded due to the regular influx of surfers from the cities, but you can still find some quiet waves if you try a few other beaches in the area and stay off the main peaks. The beachbreak at Croyde works on all tides but is best at low when it gets hollow and bowly. Definitely for advanced riders only at low tide over three-foot as the waves break very powerfully and there are some ferocious rips. Treat the locals with respect, and expect to get the best waves in the winter.

Woolacombe is a popular west facing beachbreak which works at all stages of the tide. It needs a clean swell and easterly winds to get really good. Be aware of the rip on the left hand side, and walk along the beach to find your own peak away from the crowds.

During the winter months the breaks on the south coast of Devon can go off. There are plenty of waves for everyone but when crowds become a problem the adventurous check out some of the secluded reefs. Wait for a low pressure system in the Bay of Biscay and this coast can come to life. Challaborough is a consistent mid-to-high tide left hander that picks up a fair amount of swell and is good for learners. On its day the Bantham rivermouth is a long dredging right hand barrel with frequent sections for hitting the lip. All in all a great region if you pick your day...

SOUTH COAST

The south coast has a great variety of waves between Bournemouth and Brighton. The main spots in Bournemouth are Bournemouth Pier and Boscombe Pier (and the reef!). These popular south-facing breaks work on all tides and are usually crowded whenever there's surf. Further up the coast Southbourne is a south-facing beachbreak that works on all tides, and Highcliffe is an average south-facing beachbreak which works on low to mid tide.

Further along, West Wittering and East Wittering have long stretches of southwest-facing sand and shingle beachbreak with numerous groynes that can produce decent waves. Best on southwest groundswells (which somehow wrap right around the Isle of Wight!) when northerly winds blow offshore, and best around high tide.

Brighton is a cool seaside town which is well worth a visit. There are a few spots which are generally surfed on southwest windswells during the autumn and winter months. On a big swell better quality waves break over the chalk and flint reef at The Marina which works best around mid-tide. It can get pretty crowded so is reserved for experienced surfers only. Hastings has a south-facing shingle beachbreak with a wedgy shorebreak wave next to the breakwater at the Sealife Centre. There's also a small right pointbreak at Fairlight which needs a big southwest windswell to work.

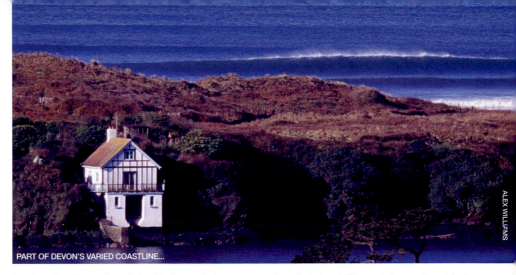

PART OF DEVON'S VARIED COASTLINE...

ALEX WILLIAMS

longboarding. On small swells head to the westerly facing beaches. St Ouen's on Jersey has a variety of spots from long walls to snappy sandbars. These spots will also hold waves up to eight feet when it's clean. If you aren't into big waves then you can find clean smaller surf at St Brelade's, which can produce fun lefts and rights. Wherever you're surfing, it's worth noting that the Channel Islands have a tidal range of up to 40 feet, so continuously shifting peaks and rip currents affect many of the breaks.

EAST COAST

One of the lesser know surf destinations in the UK, Kent gets waves when large storms blow swell down the North Sea or up the Channel. Greatstone-on-Sea is an east-facing beachbreak which occasionally offers hollow waves at high tide on a big

southwest windswell. Ramsgate is a southeast-facing beach with a couple of spots (the Harbour Wall and the Boulder Break) that occasionally work on big southwest windswells coming up the Channel. Joss Bay is another popular northeast facing spot which works on east or northeast swells. It's mostly beachbreak but there's also an area of chalk reef...

NORTH EAST

As well as being the home of Sting, Dire Straits and Newcastle Brown Ale, the North East also has some fine waves. Check out the bays around the North East's most popular surf town, Scarborough, then head along the coast to Cayton Bay – a north east facing bay with three breaks. Keep an eye on tight low pressure systems drifting northeast over the top of Scotland, sending waves and offshores down the North Sea.

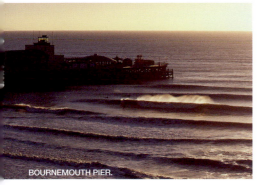

BOURNEMOUTH PIER.

CHANNEL ISLANDS

Situated 15 miles from France's Cherbourg peninsula, the Channel Islands receive the same west swells as Devon and Cornwall. The islands are great places to visit as there are waves for all standards of surfers – from gnarly big-wave reefs in winter to beachies for gentle summer swells which are ideal for

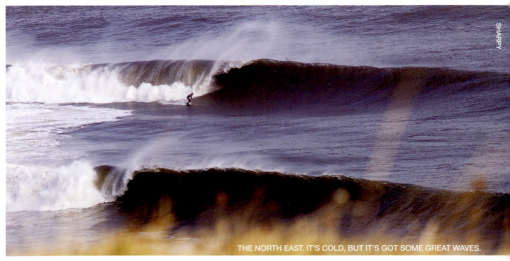

THE NORTH EAST. IT'S COLD, BUT IT'S GOT SOME GREAT WAVES.

SHARPY

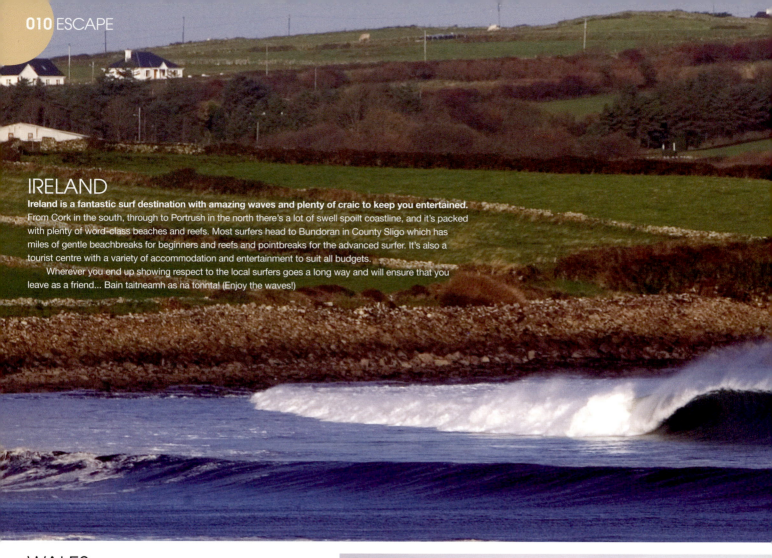

IRELAND

Ireland is a fantastic surf destination with amazing waves and plenty of craic to keep you entertained. From Cork in the south, through to Portrush in the north there's a lot of swell spoilt coastline, and it's packed with plenty of word-class beaches and reefs. Most surfers head to Bundoran in County Sligo which has miles of gentle beachbreaks for beginners and reefs and pointbreaks for the advanced surfer. It's also a tourist centre with a variety of accommodation and entertainment to suit all budgets.

Wherever you end up showing respect to the local surfers goes a long way and will ensure that you leave as a friend... Bain taitneamh as na tonnta! (Enjoy the waves!)

WALES

Wales has a lot to offer surfers, with a wide variety of breaks. The biggest and best waves come alive during the winter months, when lots of sheltered points and bays really turn on. Head to the Gower, Freshwater West, Porthcawl, or out to Pembrokeshire. Turn up at any of these spots on good days and you will see some excellent surfing. There are still plenty of semi-secret spots throughout Wales, but due to massive tidal movements and fickle winds your finger has to be on the pulse if you're to score them.

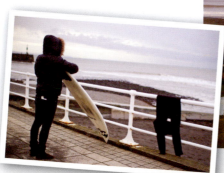

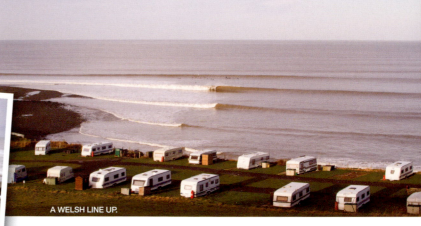

A WELSH LINE UP.

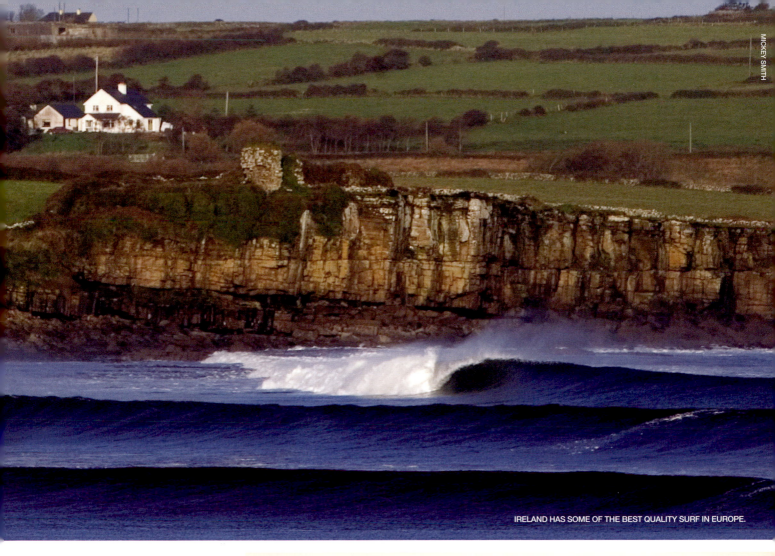

MICKEY SMITH

IRELAND HAS SOME OF THE BEST QUALITY SURF IN EUROPE.

SCOTLAND

The best thing about Scotland is that there is lots of it! Lots of space, fresh air, empty coastline and, most importantly, lots of swell.
The Western Isles receive more swell than anywhere else in Britain and have mile-after-mile of beaches, reefs and points – most of which are empty 90% of the time. Scotland also has its own North Shore which runs from Thurso to Durness and is home to many world-famous spots and some hidden gems. The Northern Isles are a surf explorer's dream, with yet more waves and deserted beaches. The east coast swells are more fickle and a little more crowded, but there are probably more surfers at Fistral on a summer's day than there are in the whole of Scotland!

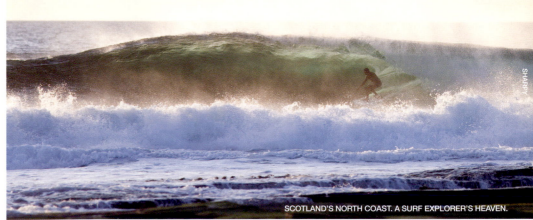

SHARPY

SCOTLAND'S NORTH COAST. A SURF EXPLORER'S HEAVEN.

TRAVEL TIPS

The journey to the perfect wave can be a long and treacherous one. Demons bent on shattering your dreams disguise themselves as airport check in clerks, baggage handlers, mad taxi drivers and hire car agents! Their job is to try and prevent you getting to your destination with your board and sanity intact, and with enough cash to survive your trip. Here are a few cunning tips to help you survive the maelstrom.

PREPARING FOR YOUR BIG TRIP!

A BASIC TRAVEL CHECK LIST:

• **Boards.** Do you have the right board(s) for the conditions you'll face?

• **Do you need wetsuits or rash vests?** Always take two pairs of boardies just in case one pair rips. And plenty of bikinis! Reef boots. They look silly, but so does sitting on the beach with reef cuts when the waves are firing.

• **Spare leashes, spare fins, fin keys and leash string.** The simple but o-so-vital things in life...

• **The right wax.** Cool water wax running off your board ain't a good look in Indo...

• **A good boardbag, packed correctly.** Don't over pack with boards, do over pack clothes/towels/wetties around your board to protect it.

• **Travel straps or racks for taxis, hire cars, buses.** Ding kit, solar resin, duck tape. Sad but true...

• **Sunscreen, total block, aloe vera aftersun, vaseline for rubs.** You'll really appreciate it when the time comes.

• **Tea tree oil.** For bites and cuts.

• **Insect repellent.** 100% jungle formula Deet works on body and bed clothes

• **Travel Insurance.** Have a copy of your policy and the number to call, and make sure you've also got the details saved somewhere safe online.

PACKING

Protection is everything. Buy a good board bag that can hold your boards – look after it and it'll last forever. Buy the right size bag for the number and type of boards you're taking and don't skimp! Coffin bags (bigger bags with a zip lid) are great and you can always bung loads of stuff in them if you're going over the baggage allowance. (Most airlines won't weigh your surfboards). If you intend to hike a lot, then go for a double bag with decent straps, as it'll be easier to carry. The most vulnerable parts of a surfboard are the nose and tail (and fixed fins, but they're pretty rare nowadays), so pad these with towels/wetties.

TAKE A SPARE BOARD!

If you want to surf big waves on your travels then make sure you've got a board that you're confident with and that can handle the additional power. Get a gun, try it out at your local break to make sure you like the way it paddles, turns etc. If you have to save up – then get on with it now! There is no substitute for the confidence you get from being happy with your equipment when you are paddling for the wave of your life!

If you only want to take one board go for something a little longer than you would normally ride and more suited to being an all rounder. It may not go so well when it's two feet, but if it gets big it won't hinder you either.

Get travel insurance that covers surfboards.

CHECKING IN

Always be polite to the check in folk as they have the ability to make your life hell!

When checking boards in at the airport always ask if they are going as part of your luggage allowance because they're so light. If you have to weigh them put your foot under the back of the boardbag to support it and take off some of the weight.

Most airline companies have cottoned on to the fact that they can make a bit of extra cash from surfers carrying boards so always check the cost before you book your ticket. Remember the golden rule: one board bag = one board. Try to avoid Iberia, KLM or American Airlines. They are really surf unfriendly and will try to charge you ridiculous amounts to take your boards.

Make sure you budget for the board taxes (it's at the airport in Hawaii), and don't take more than three boards each into Bali as they'll be taxed.

If you suspect that your board's been damaged after a flight then check it immediately and report any damage to the airline. Most airlines require that you sign an indemnity form these days, but that shouldn't exclude them from negligent damage.

Always dress well when travelling. You never know when you may get an upgrade on a flight, or need to look well presented to impress the local police in places like Indonesia.

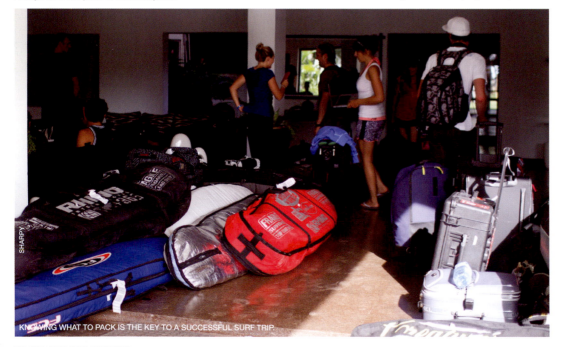

KNOWING WHAT TO PACK IS THE KEY TO A SUCCESSFUL SURF TRIP.

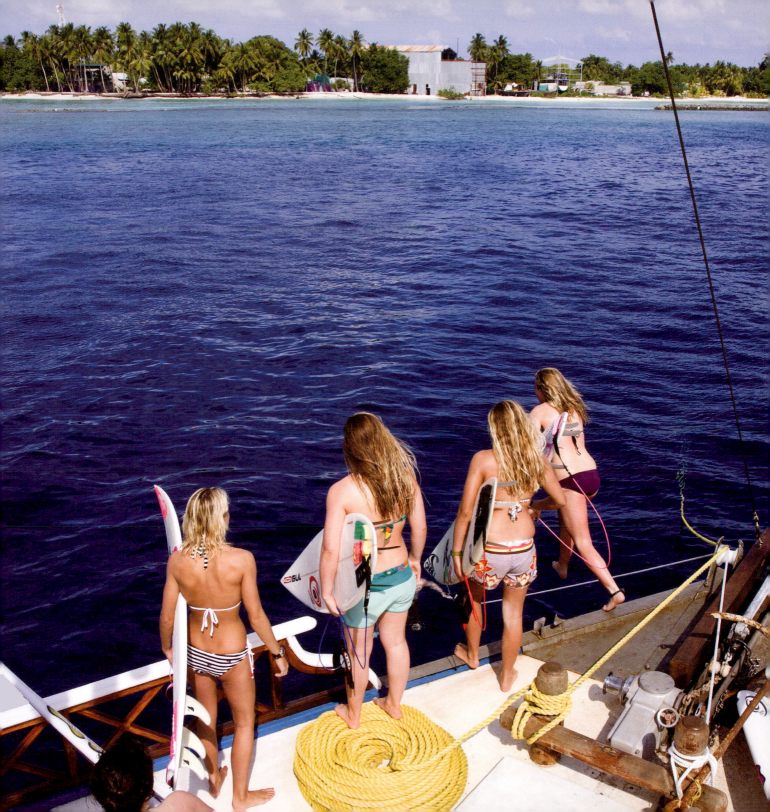

GLOSSARY

AERIAL An explosive manoeuvre where the surfer launches himself into the air, off the top of the wave.

BARREL A tubular section of a wave within which a surfer can find the meaning of life.

BACKHAND To ride with your back to the wave.

BEACHBREAK Waves that break over a sandy bottom, ideal for beginners.

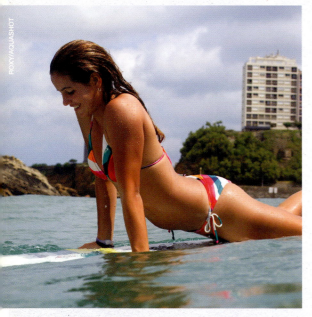

BOTTOM TURN Having dropping down the face of the wave, this is the first turn a surfer uses to set up the next move.

CLOSEOUT A wave which breaks along its length all at once, without peeling. Also

known as a straight-hander.

CARVE Cool Brit surf mag. Also a powerful turn that throws up loads of spray.

CUTBACK A manoeuvre performed on the shoulder of the wave that turns the surfer back toward the pocket.

DROP IN When a surfer takes off on a wave that someone else is already riding; a serious breach of surfing etiquette. Remember: the surfer nearest the curl has right of way.

DUCK DIVE The method used by a surfer to push his or her board under an oncoming wave while paddling out.

DING A hole in your surfboard. Often the result of dropping in!

FOREHAND To ride facing the wave.

FLOATER A manoeuvre where the surfer rides over the breaking section of the wave and free-falls down the wave's curtain.

FILTHY Extremely good.

GLASSY Clean, smooth surf conditions when there is no wind.

GNARLY An evil mutha of a wave, intent on destruction; evil conditions.

GOOFYFOOT A surfer who rides right-foot-forward.

GOING OFF! When the waves are really good, or someone's ripping.

GROMMET A young surfer with no respect for his or her elders, usually in need of some discipline!

GROUNDSWELL A swell caused by a low pressure system quite a way offshore.

GUN A long, narrow surfboard designed for riding big waves.

IMPACT ZONE The area where the waves break.

KOOK An idiot who has no idea what he or she is doing.

LEFT-HANDER A wave that breaks towards the left as seen from the lineup.

LINEUP The area where waves jack up before they break, where surfers wait.

LOCAL Someone who surfs a spot regularly, and enjoys moaning on and on about crowds.

MAL Traditional style surfboard around nine feet in length. Hang ten dude!

NAILED To get hammered by the lip of a big wave.

NATURAL FOOT A surfer who rides left-foot-forward.

OFFSHORE When the wind blows from the land to the sea, holding up the waves. The ideal wind for surfing.

ONSHORE The exact opposite. Time to head down the pub!

OVER THE FALLS The worst kind of wipeout, when you get dragged down stuck in the lip of the wave.

POINTBREAK A rock headland around which waves peel, either to the left or right.

PUMPING When the surf is going off.

POCKET The part of the wave just in front of the curl, where it's steepest.

QUIVER A selection of surf boards to suit different conditions.

RAILS The edges of a surfboard.

REEFBREAK A wave that breaks out to sea, over a slab of rock or coral. Not suitable for beginners.

RIP A dangerous current that can pull you out to sea. If you get caught in one, don't panic, but paddle across it to where the waves are breaking.

RIGHT-HANDER A wave that breaks towards the right, as seen from the lineup.

RHINO CHASER A really big board designed for charging huge waves.

ROCKER The bottom curve along the length of a surfboard.

SET A group of larger waves which come in periodically.

SICK Very good.

SHOREBREAK Where waves break close to the sand at a steep beach.

SHOULDER The sloping unbroken part of the wave ahead of the pocket.

SOUP The whitewater where a wave has just broken. Also a nice hot liquid to be consumed in large quantities after a winter session.

TUBE The same as a barrel.

WIPEOUT See nailed!

ZOO A badly crowded lineup.

ROXY/AQUASHOT

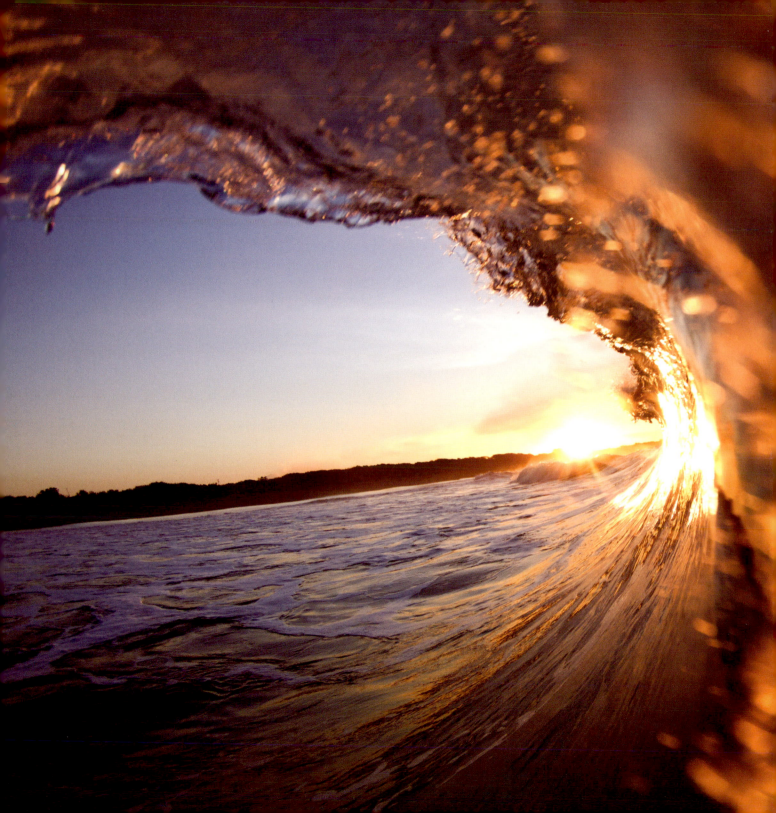

NOTES: queshten, for Jon
tell unckie Jon me know
what Duck Diveing is for
suafing

I got up this morning,
and ran to the beach,
and the surf was pumping!

SURF JOURNAL:

*I love the summer mornings
when the wind's offshore
and the surf's clean and glassy!*

surf girl Summer

Dreaming of...

sunsets cocktails summer breeze beach barbecue easy livin' laughter camping
sunrise heat sand suntan oil smell of coconut golden glow sunshine holidays good friends surf cordu-
road trips
roy lines warm summer loving

INDEX

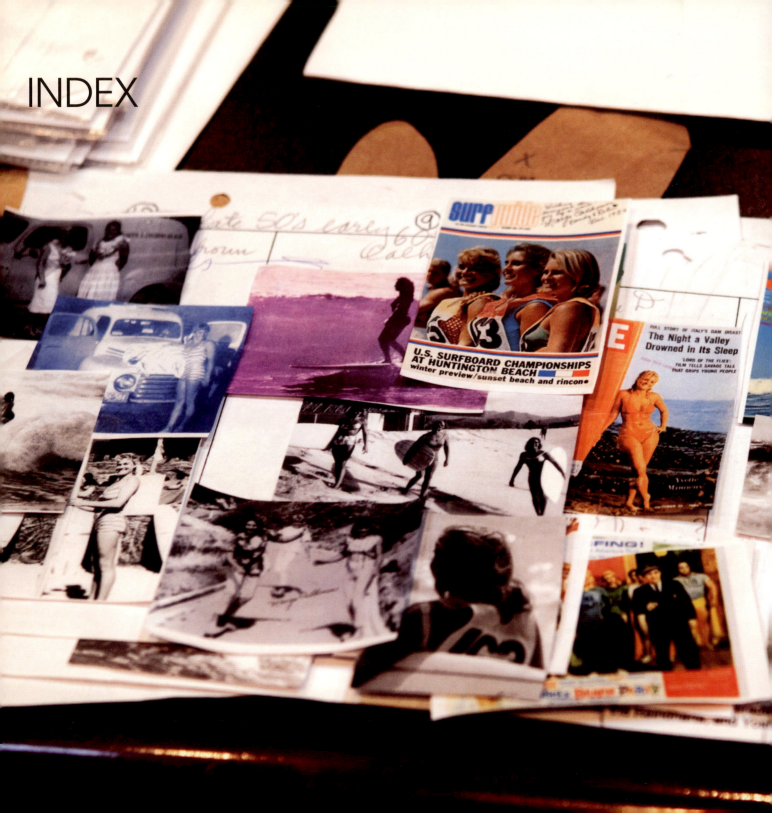

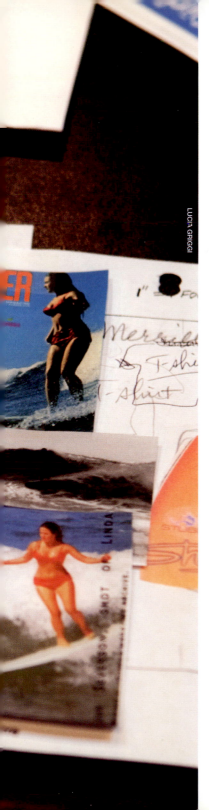

LUCIA GRIGGI

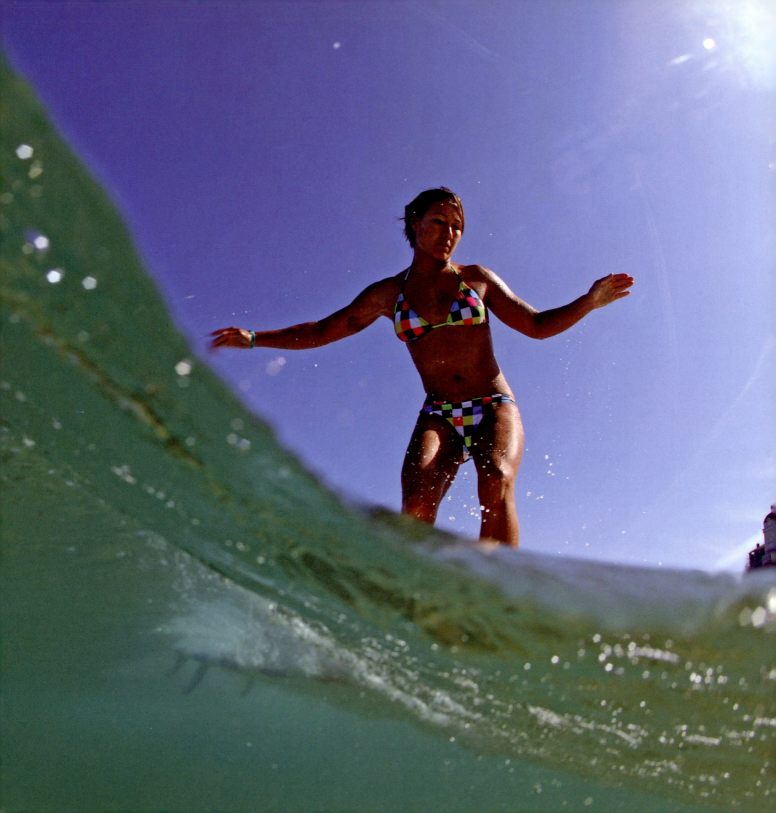

meet the
EXPERTS

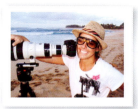

Lucia Griggi
PHOTOGRAPHER & WRITER

Lucia has long been one of SurfGirl's foremost photographers. She's equally happy shooting fashion as she is swimming out into the maelstrom of Pipeline. Over the past three years, Lucia's life has been the epitome of adventure – shooting surfing, portraits and commercial work for advertising, magazines and books – all the way from South East Asia, to the Maldives, to South Africa. And of course Hawaii.

To see more of Lucia's work go to www.luciadaniellagriggi.co.uk.

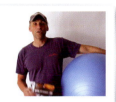

Lee Stanbury
FITNESS GURU

Lee is a qualified advanced personal trainer and instructor, and is also the strength and conditioning coach for the British Under-18 surf team, as well being a regular contributor to SurfGirl magazine.

For more information and more exercise programs check out Lee's website www.fit2surf.com

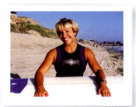

Peggy Hall
NUTRITION SPECIALIST AND YOGA INSTRUCTOR

Recognised as a leading authority on surfing wellness and fitness, Peggy Hall is an avid surfer, certified yoga instructor, surf-nutrition specialist and the creator of Yoga for Surfers – the first-ever yoga program designed specifically for surfers.

Get more info and free yoga surf stretches at www.YogaforSurfers.com.

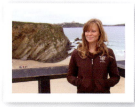

Shannon Denny
SURF JOURNALIST

Shannon grew up in landlocked Atlanta before moving to the UK, where a career in journalism has provided some amazing travel and interview opportunities. After an initial lesson in rainy Wales, she's now surfed in the US (both sides), Australia, Morocco, Bali, France and Spain, and can be found in Devon most weekends – because a girl has to earn her cream tea!

Check out her website here: www.shannondenny.com

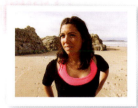

Amy Swanson
PILATES INSTRUCTOR

Amy Swanson has spent the last four years developing her own unique surf-specific Pilates programme. Through special courses run with travel companies Big Friday and Errant Surf, Amy has been able to develop her programme to suit both novice surfers and pros such as Celine Gehret.

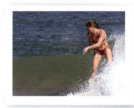

Carolyn Andrews
PERSONAL FITNESS TRAINER

A personal fitness trainer for 10 years, Carolyn is an avid surfer who recognised the huge benefits of strength and conditioning training to help improve fitness in the surf.

A contributor to SurfGirl as well as many other health and fitness magazines, Carolyn spent several years in Cornwall, personal training, teaching fitness and as a beach lifeguard, but she's now decamped to the Sunshine Coast.

Her website is full of tips, advice and exercises to help you to get fit to surf. www.surf-fit.co.uk.

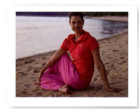

Sam McGee
YOGA TEACHER

Samantha Magee has been practicing yoga for over 10 years. She now teaches adults and children, and has developed a loyal following that includes a number of celebrity clientele.

Sam's a regular contributor to SurfGirl and Yoga Magazine and teaches regularly in studios throughout London. She is also founder of the Yamarama Yoga Wear range, www.yamarama.com.

Plus a big thanks to the surfers and coaches who contributed to the Surf Girl Handbook; Sally Fitzgibbons, Sarah Beardmore, Candice O'Donnell, Dominique Kent, Easkey Britton, Celine Gehret and Joel Gray.

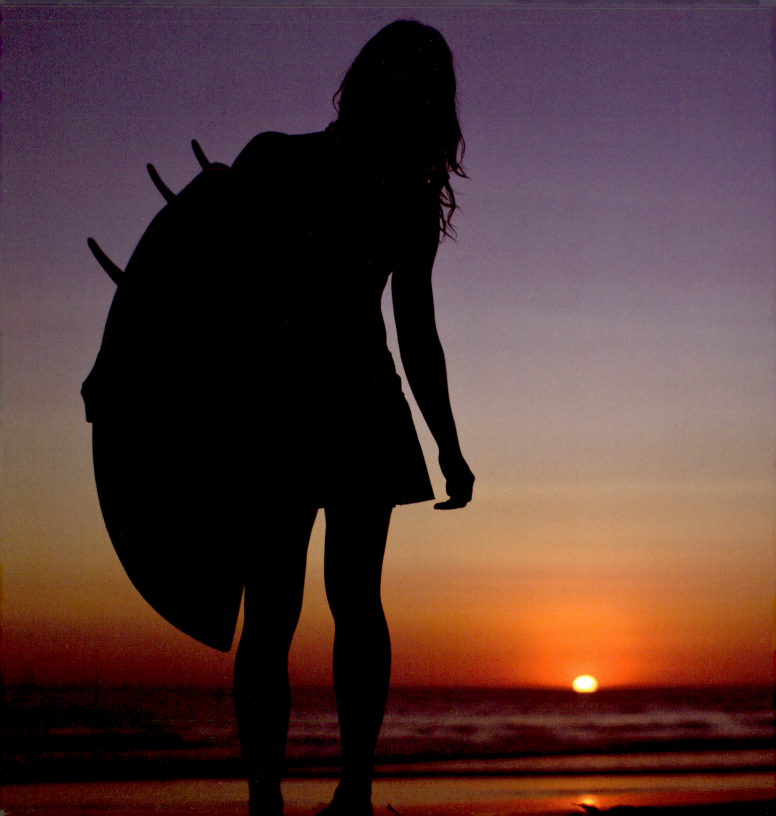